187 Excuses
Why You Are Still
Overweight

Jack G. Elder

Disclaimer

The author is not a licensed practitioner, physician, or medical professional and offers no medical diagnosis, treatments, suggestions, or counseling. Full medical clearance from a licensed physician should be obtained before beginning or modifying any diet, exercises or lifestyle program and physician should be informed of all nutritional changes.

The Author claims no responsibility to any person or entity for any liability lost or damage caused or alleged to be caused directly or indirectly because of the use, application, or interpretation of the information as presented herein. This book is for motivation and entertainment. Contact physician before starting any weight loss program.

ISBN: 9781729425794

Contents

Acknowledgments

I want to thank my editor and wife Charlene for her input on the project as well as her encouragement in our weight loss journey. Mutual support helps along the way to minimize the excuses and makes weight loss a possibility.

<u>Introduction</u>

Now before I venture further down this path of excuses, I will say there are opposing views on whether being overweight is our fault. Modern thinking says we are all victims and we are okay just the way we are. "I'm okay, you're okay." This same thinking says we should strike the word "bad" from our vocabulary stating nothing is bad because we don't want people to think they are bad and do bad things. I will admit I come from the view of a Christian senior citizen who has observed all these "new" ways of thinking and pretty much put them in a category I call "new age hooey."

I'm also of the idea that you can do all things through Christ and being overweight is not a good thing regardless whether you call fat big and beautiful. Therefore, this old fogey might have old-fashioned thinking, but it comes with theological insight and many years of observing what really works. This is about excuses, which has meaning to all of life but I'm focusing on the overweight excuses. You won't find a diet in Chapter 10; hey, there is no Chapter 10, but I've tried to sprinkle in some tips for weight loss and overcoming excuses.

This is in no way a condemnation for the overweight but my way of trying to help slow this growing epidemic. This is not to shame anyone or make them feel guilty in any way for being overweight. I know the struggle people have with weight and I just want to help each to overcome. Writers wrestle over using the word "you" as it might sound too preachy. I just want to talk to you in a friend-to-friend dialogue and say I'm hoping when you see the excuses you will see yourself in them and want to lose the weight. I want you to have every opportunity to live a healthy life.

Also, I want to mention that in this book of excuses to losing weight, I am using the words, "diet," "weight loss diet," "weight loss," or "weight loss journey" in generic terms. I'm not suggesting any particular diet or non-diet method of losing weight. I'm just saying I feel weight loss is important and whatever method you find to get the weight off is great. Every method requires something from you, and although the methods may change, the need to quit making excuses, the need to do something is common to all weight loss methods, thus, the need to quit making excuses and start making changes.

Chapter 1

Excuses, Excuses

If you've been dieting as long as I have, you have probably been on almost every diet imaginable, as most of us weight challenged folks have, and along the way, you have told yourself plenty of lies. See if any of these sound familiar. I'm sure you have heard broken cookies don't have any calories. Cookies eaten in secret don't add fat. These cookies are only one bite each. I'll just walk more today if I have a cookie. I'll start my diet tomorrow. I'd rather eat a cookie than a carrot. Some people are so good at dieting they finish a 14-day diet in 4 hours. (Don't laugh, because you've probably been there). Fat is good for you, so eat a butter stick. They say peanuts are good for you, so I eat a jar a day. Well, I have to eat, don't I? I'll just take one bite. These would be funny if not for the fact we are talking about our health.

Some of the excuses come from myths about dieting. Yes, some diets are extreme and people have said some bad things about weight loss because of it. I found some synonyms for weight loss on the internet and some of them promote the idea dieting is just horrible. How about some of these: starve, eat sparingly, deny oneself, not eat, go hungry, famish, impoverish, refrain, debase, dwindle, and impair just to name a few. No wonder dieting and weight loss gets a bad rap. Some of the excuses come out of this philosophy, but dieting doesn't have to be any of this negative thinking.

Let's Define Excuse

Before we launch into any specific excuses let's see what an excuse is. The dictionary defines excuse as, "reason, or explanation put forward to defend or justify a fault or offense." The Urban dictionary says, "They are tools of incompetence, used to build monuments of nothingness, and those who specialize in them seldom accomplish anything." That's a little more brutal.

However you define the word, an excuse usually is something negative you use as a defense against doing something positive. In our case here, an excuse about weight loss. I believe weight loss is good, positive, and right. An excuse is why you don't believe such a statement. Some excuses are just silly even said as a joke, such as, "If you put a crouton on your sundae instead of a cherry, it counts as a salad." Humorous maybe, but excuses are not funny. Weight loss is a serious endeavor and failing is the easy way out most people take. The easiest way to write off weight loss is with an excuse. Have you heard of a lame excuse? All excuses are lame and merely allow you to limp through life. Some are just hopelessly terminal.

Progress or Excuse

With weight loss, there are only two options—yes or no. I could say it another way if I said there are two options—progress or excuse. Now I'm not saying everyone should be on a weight loss diet. There are all kinds of diets, such as disease related, weight gain diets, and other diets, even non-diets. I'm not a doctor, at least not a medical doctor, so I'm not going to discuss medical diets here with this caveat, some medical diets could go away with weight loss.

Anyway, if you are the average person who is overweight, from a few pounds to many pounds, then this book addresses many of the excuses associated with weight loss. I've personally experienced many of the excuses; in fact, this could be my list. For the weight loss challenged person, we face the never-ending trial of using excuses in an attempt to solve our weight loss problems—doesn't work. You will make no progress with excuses. The two are opposites. Either you make progress or you make excuses. My suggestion is to toss the excuses and start making your weight loss journey a monumental accomplishment in your life.

Healthy and Excuses Don't Fit Together

If you want to be heathy, you have to give up one thing—your excuses.

There are two subjects, which don't match, health and excuses. I'm sometimes surprised at how many people don't consider health a high priority. I guess I shouldn't be surprised. The pharmaceutical commercials fill the TV with promoting their latest pill or procedure. Have a problem take a pill.

First, these thoughts have numbed us to health problems, and second we have seemingly replaced trying to be healthy with using medical methods and a pill. The incidents of obesity and even morbid obesity tells me people don't care. In fact, not caring is one of their excuses, which we will lcok at later. However, we thwart any attempt to be healthy through diet by giving excuses.

By the way, obesity is defined as an accumulated of body fat possibly resulting in a negative effect on their health. If your bodyweight is at least 20% higher than it should be or your Body Mass Index (BMI) is between 25 and 29.9, you are obese. Morbid obesity means being more than 100 pounds overweight or a BMI greater than 40. Morbid obesity is a medical condition in which excess body fat has an adverse effect on health.

We still smoke tobacco in this nation in spite of all the dire predictions, smoking is going to harm the body in so many ways. Therefore, I guess it goes without saying cutting out sugar is not going over very well either.

I delivered Meals on Wheels when I was in California. I met many people who had put their health on the back burner and were now in serious health trouble. Now I'm not implying losing weight fixes all health problems. However, I'm saying we all know the health problems caused by excess weight. So eliminating one potential hindrance to your health is big, and any excuse to completing the goal is a way not to reach the goal.

Excuses Are Cheap

You can get a hundred excuses for a nickel, maybe a couple of pennies on sale. Everyone has heard the saying talk is cheap; well this is the same quote with slightly different words. Excuses are just empty talk, clouds without rain. They don't carry weight and no one believes them. Why do we give excuses when people know they aren't true?

Yes, there might be a time when an excuse is a good reason, but mostly excuses are just empty reasons. I guess there is something in our heads scrambling for a reason, good or bad, for our poor decisions. An excuse doesn't cost you anything today but your health.

The opposite of giving an excuse is not giving an excuse. Instead of trying to justify your poor decisions, reverse your thinking and starting seeing some good. In theological terms, it means to repent—change your thinking. The best way to see results is to start making results happen. Get moving on your weight loss journey—today. Next month when there is progress, you'll see the excuses were just self-lies blocking your results. You won't make any excuse for winning.

Excuses – I've Got a Million of Em

"I got a million of em" is an old famous Jimmy Durante line. I'm a senior but you might not know who Jimmy Durante was. Popularly known as "Schnozzola," he was an American singer, actor, comedian, and pianist starting out in the vaudeville days of the 20's. I've also heard countless excuses, and I have made countless excuses in my weight loss journey. By the way, the weight loss journey for overweight or obese people is a never-ending journey, even if you reach goal. I don't think I can list a million excuses but it's surprising how many weight loss excuses are out there. Okay, maybe not surprising. Do a search on "diet excuses" and you'll get 11,100 hits (at time I looked). Why are we always looking for an excuse for our failures?

The First Excuse

"9 And the LORD God called unto Adam, and said unto him, Where *art* thou? 10 And he said, I heard thy voice in the garden, and I was afraid, because I *was* naked; and I hid myself. 11 And he said, Who told thee that thou *wast* naked? Hast thou eaten of the tree, whereof I commanded thee that thou shouldest not eat? 12 And the man said, The woman whom thou gavest *to be* with me, she gave me of the tree, and I did eat" (Genesis 3:9-12).

You can see excuses have been around a long time. When Adam ate of the forbidden fruit, his excuse was the woman God gave him made him take the fruit. Sometimes excuses come off as blame. Something happened to make me do it. Remember Flip Wilson, yes another old timer, who said, "The devil made me do it." He was probably closer to the truth, but still there is always a point where you have a choice. Adam had a choice and still took the fruit. He could have turned the fruit down, but he chose to blame God for giving him the woman instead. Make the right choice and you don't have to make an excuse.

Moses Had Plenty of Excuses

Exodus Chapter 4 begins with "And Moses answered and said." From there he gave God one excuse after another. What will they say? I'm not a good speaker. Finally, the Bible records, "So the anger of the LORD was kindled against Moses." Moses' excuses finally angered God. God didn't however give up on Moses. God said He would help him. Fortunately, Moses did what God told him and what Moses thought he couldn't do, He did, and he became a mighty leader of God's people.

You can make excuses to God. He isn't going to reject you, because Jesus already took your rejection. You can overcome the excuses and turn them into victories. As God told Moses, "I will teach you what you shall do." With God's help, you can do anything.

Where Do Excuses Come From?

Where do excuses come from? The devil made me do it. The devil can play a role in your making excuses because they come from your view of life and yourself. We all have excuses about various mistakes and awkward situations in our life. Our excuses come from false beliefs, which may have risen in early childhood about what other people might have said or fears about things in life. They come from beliefs, which say we don't deserve anything, or we tried and failed at everything. Excuses often come from a false notion of "can't." Maybe you have never actually tried something, but you turned it into a "can't." You might say I don't like mushrooms for example, but you have never tried to eat mushrooms. Maybe you don't like to do certain activities such as selling, so you turned your dislike into a "can't"—an excuse.

Many people have told excuses so long and so many times, they're used to taking the excuse way out. What would your life be like if you just never made another excuse? You would begin to find a way. You would succeed where before you failed. Your life would be positive rather than negative. You would be happy rather than sad or mad. The excuse comes from within you. Turn your excuse into success by just turning it around from no to yes.

An Excuse Is a Lie

Excuses are lies we tell ourselves so it won't be our fault. Put the blame elsewhere, not my responsibility, or is it? You are the only one who can live your life. Your life is yours, your responsibility to manage each day. You will make mistakes. You will have successes. Accepting both is living within yourself.

Some excuses are marginally good reasons. When you get older, some activities you no longer desire to do. I don't care to jog anymore. However, there are older people who still do. I watched a 100-year-old woman run the 100-meter dash and shatter the record for her age group. Another 100-year-old ran a marathon. We actually can do more than we think we can do. Excuses just limit our potential.

Being overweight also limits your potential, and not wanting to change, certainly limits what you can be. You are putting up barriers in your life by your excuses. It is one matter to overcome the obstacles, but when you put them there yourself, I call that self-defeating and dare I say—stupid. You can do more than you think you can, so don't make excuses about it.

Excuses Are Self-Lies

You may be speaking your excuse to someone, but you are simply lying to yourself. Lies are false statements, untrue comments, and fabricated falsehoods. There are cases when you don't realize you are telling a lie when you make an excuse. Sometimes you think you are just uttering a fact or observation. I can't diet. Is it true? No. You can diet.

It's not good to tell someone a lie, but making an excuse is telling yourself a lie. Listening to these self-lies will just further deceive you into failure. Tell yourself the truth. Don't make excuses. If you really can't do something, then don't try. If you can't jog, then don't jog. You don't have to if you don't want to. I don't jog. I can jog some but I don't like to and I don't want to jog. Tell the truth and it won't become an excuse.

Liar, liar pants on fire.

<u>An Excuse Is Self-Destruction</u>

The only one an excuse hurts is you. Now if you are obese and you excuse yourself from losing weight, then your excuse will eventually hurt others. However, it starts with you. You are your own decision maker. Whatever you decide affects you directly. This applies to life as well as weight loss. Putting off weight loss is neglecting yourself. An excuse is just self-neglect—self-destruction.

I can say this because I have no ulterior motive in trying to get you to diet if you are obese or overweight. I'm not selling you any supplements or my latest book—yet. I'm hoping the love comes through to you. As Saint John said, "Beloved, I pray that you may prosper in all things and be in health, just as your soul prospers" (3 John 1:2 NKJV). I pray you will live a long healthy life. I'm concerned about your health if you are overweight or obese. You can take this one good step for yourself. Don't let an excuse keep you from a happy life. Weight loss by itself isn't going to make you happy, but losing weight goes a long way toward happiness.

<u>An Excuse or a Reason</u>

Did you give an excuse or a reason? Sometimes you can't discern the difference. In the definition of excuse many use the word reason—"a reason or explanation put forward to defend or justify a fault or offense." Therefore, an excuse is a reason to justify a failure. A reason is "a cause, explanation, or justification for an action or event." A reason is just telling the truth about an action. Why can't you walk? An excuse—I don't like to walk. Reason—there's thunder and lightning out there.

I know there is a fine line between a reason and an excuse. An excuse is why you can't when you really can. A reason is why you can't when you really can't. I have a friend whose wife just had knee replacement. She has a temporary reason why she can't get out and walk. Before she had the surgery, her knee hurt too bad to walk much. However, when her knee heals, she will get out and walk again.

Therefore, when people give an excuse, they are covering their failure. When they give a reason, they are explaining the present situation and not trying to get out of something. Excuse – not good. Reason – good, with qualifications.

Are There Any Good Excuses?

If you do a Google search on "good excuses," you will get 339,000 hits (at the time I looked). You will see articles such as 15 good excuses for getting out of work. These excuses are pure lies, such as you had an accident and survived without a scratch but totaled the car, so you need to get the car fixed. Well, if you totaled the car, you had better show up to work with a different car. Excuses such as these are lies. There are no good excuses. They are all bad excuses.

We don't have a good excuse to keep us from our appointed weight loss journey. I hope you aren't one of those who would tell a lie to your boss to get out of work. I also hope you are not one of those who would tell yourself a lie to get out of losing the fat you're carrying around town. There are a few valid reasons why not to diet, but there are no good excuses. So trash the excuse and set your chubby tummy free.

Know Your Excuses

Know your excuses. Excuses are sneaky. They are like calories, you know those tiny creatures living in your closet and stitching your clothes a bit tighter each night. Everyone has excuses. Excuses somehow salve the pain of failure. Well, I knew I couldn't do it anyway. We know our weaknesses and know when we pull back from something. We know what we fear out there in the unknown. Look carefully at those excuses and overcome them, even if that's not always easy.

The Apostle Paul had weaknesses and wanted the Lord to remove them, but He wouldn't. God said the way to overcome is through God's grace—it's sufficient. "**9** And he said unto me, My grace is sufficient for thee: for my strength is made perfect in weakness. Most gladly therefore will I rather glory in my infirmities, that the power of Christ may rest upon me. **10** Therefore I take pleasure in infirmities, in reproaches, in necessities, in persecutions, in distresses for Christ's sake: for when I am weak, then am I strong" (2 Corinthians 12:9-10).

Know your weaknesses and turn those into **No** weaknesses through grace, God's unmerited favor, and power given as a gift to you. There is a way out.

<u>Well Excuse Me</u>

You probably heard the old Steve Martin line—"well, excuuuuuuse me." I know many of these excuses will hit home. What do you do when you speak a weight loss excuse? Maybe you ignore the statement, laugh at yourself, question what you said, or maybe you confront the problem. Ignoring and laughing won't help anything. However, looking for the solution for the immensity of the obstacle will solve the problem without excuses.

Have you heard the verse, speaking the truth in love? Some people use the verse to abuse others. They don't get the love part. As a weight challenged person you might say, "I can't," then you need to look for some options to change what you say to "I can." Speak love to yourself.

Maybe you don't want help. So "well, excuuuuuuse me," or another one I've heard, "well excuse me for living." No, I'm not going to excuse you for making an excuse. To be a real friend isn't just agreeing with an excuse, but assisting beyond the limited boundaries in which you are trapped. So excuse me if I don't accept your excuse.

Excuses Are the Easy Way Out

Fail a weight loss diet, take the easy way out, and don't go on a weight loss diet again. Just get fat and suffer the consequences. Instead of eating healthy, just take the easy way out and eat all the fast food you want. No one loses weight by taking the easy way.

There are two roads to success. One is easy and one is hard. The easy way is to do nothing. The hard way is to make changes. The easy way is to make excuses. The hard way is to make solutions. I don't want to make weight loss dieting seem as if you're taking a hard road but dieting isn't easy or everyone would be thin.

Theodore Wilson said, "Nothing in the world is worth having or worth doing unless it means effort, pain, difficulty...I have never in my life envied a human being who led an easy life. I have envied a great many people who led difficult lives and led them well." Weight loss is a challenge, but worth the cost. Anything worth having is worth pursuing. So don't take the easy way and do nothing. Instead, take the hard way, and turn it into the easy way.

Excuses Don't Burn Calories

I thought this saying was right on the money, particularly for us weight loss challenged. A calorie is a unit of heat used to indicate the amount of energy foods will produce in the human body. The body saves excess calories as fat. Stored fat is what we have to reduce if we are to reduce our weight. We also need to keep from storing any more fat.

We need a calorie deficit in order to lose. What calories we eat minus the calories we use results in a deficit or a surplus. To obtain a deficit requires a weight loss diet, which provides fewer calories to eat than we use, in addition maybe some exercise to burn extra calories. Calories in and calories out. Maybe overly simplistic, however the results have to be an overuse of calories to force your body to obtain calories stored as fat.

Although, the theory isn't quite so simple since the body doesn't always cooperate. Regardless, making excuses has zero help in getting a calorie deficit. Approximate 3500 calories used above what the body needs will lead us to lose one pound. Excuses make no difference in the weight loss equations except to throw barriers up to the weight loss process. Burn the calories, and dump the excuses.

<u>Excuse = Failure</u>

Failure comes to those who make excuses. An excuse is just another failure waiting to happen. You impress no one with excuses. One saying is excuses are the nails, which build the house of failure. Winners use failure as motivation, while losers use failure as an excuse. Nothing comes of excuses. Failure isn't failure until failure becomes an excuse. Excuses just give us permission to fail. You are excusing yourself from doing what you know is best for you.

Weight loss is difficult, and there are often setbacks. Like the saying, falling down is not failure. Refusing to get up is. If you quit after one fail, you will never succeed at weight loss. A good weight loss chart is not a smooth line down the graph, but jagged. However, the results will be good. If you weigh every day, then the weight might not look good on a particular day. Despair not, just keep losing weight.

There's no failure in weight loss unless you quit. I hope there will come a time in your weight loss journey where you run out of excuses, and just get with the program. The sooner the better. Nothing good comes from excuses, unless you finally hear yourself giving them, the light bulb turns on, and you refuse to make any more excuses. Excuses = failure. No excuses = success.

Three steps you can take when you fail. First, don't accept failure. Second, learn from failure. Third, don't make an excuse. Edison failed some 1000 times before he got the light bulb right. He didn't accept failure, but he learned from each roadblock and didn't make excuses. Each failure should teach as more about what doesn't work. Weight loss is a learning process. We all fail at times, but we should learn something from our failure and move on to victory.

What's Your Excuse?

I still make an excuse now and then. However, the goal is to get better at eliminating the excuses.

Excuses never profit. They are like a leak in the dam. They start small and soon there is a catastrophe afoot. The best way to avoid making excuses is simply not to make excuses. What are your excuses? Have you thought about them and their hindrance to your progress?

Most people don't want to admit they are making excuses. If there were an Excuses Anonymous, the first item on the list would be to admit you make excuses. We all do. Whether we actually speak them to someone or we just keep them in our heads, we have a lineup of excuses ready for any potential failure. No one likes failure so naturally there will be an excuse ready when you slipup.

However, weight loss excuses tend to cause the failure. The excuse perpetuates failure. Let's get the obesity rate down in America. Let's make promises not excuses.

I've noticed in older age we can think up more excuses. Maybe we older people have just heard so many. However, we don't have the right to spend our mature years doing nothing except making excuses for doing nothing.

"He that is good for making excuses is seldom good for anything else" Benjamin Franklin.

"If you really want to do it, you do it. There are no excuses" Bruce Nauman.

Excuses just postpone success. Dieters who make excuses will just excuse themselves to fail. An excuse is a failure. Are there legitimate excuses? Perhaps, but fewer than you might think. Excuses are counter-productive.

An excuse is just saying what you think about the issue. You don't want to do something so you make an excuse. Like Nike says, "Just do it," and I add "Enough with the excuses."

Chapter 2

Eating Excuses

The excuses in this section are primarily about the eating aspect of your weight loss diet. This is perhaps the most important part and the bulk of the excuses. You can probably get away without exercise, but you can't get away without eating. Everyone eats but to lose weight you have to make some special adjustments, thus you're open for excuses.

Excuse 1 - I Don't Know Where to Start

The whole diet landscape is vast with so much data and so many diets, where do you start. You might want to lose some weight, but you really don't have a starting point. There is so much information out there in cyberspace a common question might be where to begin this weight loss journey.

Most people hear about a diet on TV, from a colleague, or friend, buy a book, and just jump in and start doing the plan. Maybe you scanned the diet section in the local bookstore and didn't know which book to buy. I know I occasionally look through the section for the latest. There are many famous diets such as Atkins, South Beach, Mediterranean, Weight Watchers, Jenny Craig, and so on. Each one has various pros and cons. Each handles the dieting differently. Not every diet is for everyone. Therefore the reason why there are so many diets.

I really suspect few, if any, will read this having never been on a weight loss diet before. I also suspect when you look through the diet books at the bookstore, you will flip back to about chapter 10 and see what you get to eat. If you are between diets as so many are, then make a list of what you want out of a diet. Do you want organic, vegan, non-dairy, etc.? Do you want menus? Do you want support? Do you want exercise guidance as well? Do you want flexibility or more restriction? Are you mainly interested in eating clean or do you have a medical issue? Maybe you don't want a conventional diet, perhaps even an anti-diet. Everything you need is out there, for your choosing.

My suggestion is once you have your diet wants list complete, then begin searching for one which fulfills your needs. Is your list primarily, low carb, vegan, low fat, or one of the other many categories? Start your research now. Websites such as freedieting.com are a good resource to research diets. Find a diet, which interests you and read the pros and cons, buy the book, and start the diet. There are many alternatives to the diet in the book. Maybe you want more counsel and want to get away from the standard diets. There are plenty of options. The main point here is just start a weight loss diet. Nothing happens until you start. Nothing will change until you start. You can't eat the elephant until you take the first bite. I don't recommend elephant.

Excuse 2 – I'm Always Hungry

Yeah, me too. "But wait"... What do you mean by hungry? Do you mean you're starving, or do you mean you could eat more? People define being hungry or hunger differently. One definition is "Hunger is defined as the uneasy or painful sensation caused by a recurrent or involuntary lack of food." Another definition, "a feeling of discomfort or weakness caused by lack of food, coupled with the desire to eat." Finally, "hunger is a feeling experienced when the glycogen level of the liver falls below a certain point, usually followed by a desire to eat."

There is lots of information on being truly hungry and "false" hunger on the internet. It's a far bigger subject than I can handle here.

Weight loss dieting, by definition, means to eat less than your body wants in order to use fat stores. Something has to go in order to lose. Yes, you must lose something in what you have been eating in order to lose weight. Some diets will say follow their diet and you will never be hungry.

For example, *The Appetite Solution: Lose Weight Effortlessly and Never Be Hungry Again*. Reviewers weren't so pleased with the idea. However, I'm not here to bash diets, but point out having dieted for many years, I don't think never being a little hungry is possible.

I think this is a total excuse to say I'm always hungry so I don't diet. A big chicken salad will fill you up. A large bowl of chicken vegetable soup will fill you up. There are good healthy weight loss meals that will knock off the hunger at least for a while. Toss in a couple mid meal snacks and you'll sail through the day.

You've probably been overeating for a long time now and your body is overweight and needs more calories to keep running. Your body gets use to levels of calories and wants them—now. Changing the intake is going to make the body scream for a while until figuring out this is all I'm going to get so I better make the best of less.

I saw a show the other night where the person was eating over 10,000 calories a day. Course she was 777 pounds. A person such as this or even a person 50 pounds overweight has been used to eating more than they should.

Instead of hungry, you might be thirsty. Have a glass of water, a cup of tea or a mug of coffee. Have a low-calorie snack such as carrots, celery, or a few grapes.

Cutting back to the right size portions will cause a bit of hunger. My experience with being overweight is my body always wanted more anyway. I was always a little "hungry." You must have a strong reason to diet, which will take you through the "meantime."

Excuse 3 - I Can't Figure Out What to Eat Each Day

Okay, a new eating plan, and a new menu might be daunting. Nevertheless, you have figured out what to eat each meal so far in your life, so this is an adaptation of your normal eating. Many diets have daily menus or sample menus to give you an idea of meals to eat. Some even have a week's worth of menus. I use to set up a spreadsheet with what we would eat each meal, very time-consuming to say the least. However, it worked and made making a grocery list easier. Once you make one week of meals then next week you use the same menu and make a few changes for variety.

If you are going on the weight loss trip without a formal plan, then take some time to get some meals planned out. Look for main dish recipes and sides and put together some meals. Rotate them and if you don't like something, change the meal.

For weight loss dieting, the simpler the better. You might even have the same meal for each day. Nothing wrong with having a chicken salad for lunch every day. Hey, you just took care of seven meals, only 14 plus snacks to go. Find meals you really like and then stick to them.

Make easy preparation meals for breakfast, such as a protein smoothie, or eggs, toast, and grapefruit. Starting is a little tough but once you get a few days figured out, the menu becomes easier. Easy makes the weight loss trip more enjoyable.

Excuse 4 - I Can't Afford To Diet

When I hear this, I think of some of the diets I've been on were costly. I remember the first time I went shopping to Whole Foods with my diet food list and our normal budget for a week's groceries for two was $80. The bill totaled over $200 dollars. That was hard to swallow and consequently the last week we were on that diet.

No, I'm not going to say you can't afford not to diet. I hate when sales people make those statements. When you are on a fixed budget, your food is a major cost and you can't spend more. However, you can work around this excuse.

Of course, going out to eat is more expensive also. Some people go out several times a week. Figure the cost of dining out into your diet and food is much more affordable. However, when we talk diet, we aren't necessarily talking healthy. There's no guarantee if you eat a healthy diet, weight loss will follow. On a strictly technical level, the weight loss is not a result of eating "healthier" food but in eating smart and eating less for the time being. People can lose weight on diets composed primarily of donuts; yes there is a donut diet, however, I don't recommend going on the donut diet.

Weight loss happens when you take in fewer calories from any type of food than you use. Most people try to add healthy into their weight loss diet. You certainly don't want to eat unhealthy, but add more fruits, veggies, and less processed food. If you go organic, free range, nondairy, gluten-free, sugar-free, low carb, and soy free, recognize this is going to cost more.

Those options you can work into your diet as you go along. Substitute your low nutrition diet for more high nutrition foods. With careful planning, you can meet your food budget and still lose weight.

Excuse 5 - I Can't Afford To Eat Healthy

I remember the first time I went on a "healthy" diet. After my first week's food bill, my conclusion was eating healthy is too expensive.

What many think eating healthy means is eating organic which is more expensive. Meat is much more expensive when range fed, etc.—probably three times as much. ($1.99 a pound at Walmart for chicken and $5.99 a pound free range.) A 2013 study from Harvard School of Public Health found eating a healthy diet (rich in fruits, vegetables, fish, and nuts) cost about $1.50 more per day per person than eating an unhealthy diet (the kind full of processed foods and refined grains). My observation is the cost is a bit higher, because healthy does cost more, therefore you have to choose wisely.

Some stores are less expensive than others are. Trader Joe's, for example, has more value priced items. Frozen is sometimes cheaper. Vegetables in season are less expensive. Watch for sales. Get there early and find meat reduced. You aren't going to eat as much on a weight loss diet. You aren't going to eat expensive desserts and pastries. You can cut the budget and phase in more healthy choices when you can. Don't let cost of healthy be an excuse to losing your weight.

No, I'm not going to say you can't afford not to eat healthy.

Excuse 6 - I Don't Know What's Healthy?

What healthy food is can be hard to figure out, which could be a big problem. This topic could be a whole book, or at least a large chapter. I remember when Hostess advertised their cupcakes as the Hostess Filled Muscle Builders. Someone once said if they advertise the food on TV, it probably isn't healthy. Of course, generalizations are not always true.

There are many experts out there saying what healthy is and is not. For every food, there are expert pros and cons. Manufacturers will never say their food is unhealthy. Many are jumping on some "healthy" bandwagons and picking out one idea the public wants to hear and cheer it on such as Cheerios are gluten-free.

Some manufacturers are trying to be healthier as the demand for healthy foods rises. Even fruits and vegetables have had health scares however, such as Romaine lettuce for example. Moreover, if they aren't organic, experts say they are unhealthy. Therefore, you are right because sometimes deciding if food is healthy is hard. Some say if the food has a nutrition label, beware.

Here's an example of pros and cons of any food item. Is there anything bad about broccoli? Even the most venerated of vegetables has serious health issues. Just do a Google search on broccoli. You'll find such headlines as "toxic broccoli." This is what makes deciding what food is healthy so difficult. Even sugar free foods have to replace the sugar with something that tastes good, either fat or artificial sweeteners.

You have to decide who you can trust to tell you if something is healthy or not. You may have limited finances and have to make compromises. You may not like some so-called healthy food, such as I hate fish. Many say avoid the inside aisles of the grocery store where the processed foods are located. Vegans will say no meat, where some diets are mostly meat. I think God designed the body to handle many problems in our diet. Do the best you can, but don't let this be an excuse.

Excuse 7 - The Recipes Are Too Complicated

To me, recipes become complicated by the kinds of hardware you need, the number and kinds of ingredients, and the preparation time. I've seen some recipes with over 30 ingredients. I'm always seeing some gadget on TV, which is supposed to make cooking easier or faster—a new pan or slicer. "Just set it and forget it." Charlene says I can't put it on the counter. I don't know how many "laborsaving" devices are now in storage in the basement.

One point about recipes I find frustrating is they may call for just a little of one ingredient such as one tablespoon of tomato paste. You go to the grocery store and buy the smallest container of tomato paste you can get, use once and the rest just sits in the refrigerator until you have to throw it out. I hate to waste stuff, and I'll probably never make the recipe again.

Some diets get on a certain ingredient kick. I've traveled all over two counties to try to find one ingredient. I want to say the diet asked for Macadamia oil, and when I found it, the ingredient was far too expensive for my budget.

When dieting you will probably use mostly one meat type such as chicken. Find recipes for putting variety in chicken. A quick online search and you will find hundreds of easy recipes. Chicken is a good candidate for the crock-pot.

Spices you can use over time if they are not too exotic. Usually, you have to use fresh spices shortly or they go bad. I like fewer ingredients. Of course, I very seldom cook, but Charlene will agree. Many recipes on the internet have five ingredients or less. Maybe if you love to cook, you'll branch out into recipes that are more complicated.

Excuse 8 - I've Always Eaten this way

How's that working out for you? If you are overweight, not good I suspect. I think we all have favorite foods and meals we had when we were children. My mom fixed a good Spam hash. Now I don't eat Spam. We had meat and potatoes and easy to prepare casseroles. I don't remember the last time I had a casserole. Tuna casserole makes me gag. My Mom never fixed fish because she and I hated fish. We might have had a roast for Sunday, which Mom left cooking on low until church ended. We hardly ever went out to eat.

Some foods we love have certain meanings for us. We often had Pizza on Friday fun nights when our kids were growing up. As Bob Dylan sang, "Times they are a changin'." What we ate growing up might have been okay but now those foods cause us to put on the pounds.

If you are overweight and want to lose the weight, then you are just going to have to make changes to the way you eat. First, eat healthy. Second, eat smaller portions. If the way you've always eaten is healthy, then good for you. However, for us weight challenged folk, we didn't eat so healthy, and I suspect there are changes on the horizon.

I know we've made a number of changes in order to get our weight off. We have to bypass the "all you can eat" places, and that's how we have to roll. The benefits of weight loss far surpass the desire to eat fattening foods. As we say, eating has to change or the weight won't.

Excuse 9 - I Don't Like Vegetables

Then you aren't going to be much of a dieter. Vegetables should be a large part of a healthy diet for everyone because they are low in calories. However, doing a search on "I hate vegetables" there are many people who actually hate vegetables. I'm not sure what else you can eat besides meat and still help you lose weight. I suspect most of your food comes from boxes. This is a serious problem because most diets recommend filling up at least half of your plate with vegetables.

Part of this is just an excuse to stay away from dieting. In reading the blogs and comments on people who hate vegetables, I found they don't hate all vegetables. Some they don't like because of their texture. Charlene for the longest time would not eat re-fried beans saying they were mushy beans but she will eat them now. She still doesn't like lima beans for the same reason. She grew up disliking the greens except for spinach. I don't like eggplant and not too crazy about the greens either. Most people don't like certain vegetables. Do you remember President Bush and his dislike for broccoli?

Vegetables are certainly good for you. They fill you up with nutrient dense fuel and little calories. 200 calories worth of broccoli will fill a grocery bag compared to one donut.

There is a large variety of vegetables. There are over 20,000 species of edible plants. Try some new ones. Keep an open mind when you try a new veggie. Go back and visit ones you thought you didn't like as a youngster. Maybe you didn't like the looks of them as a child so thought you didn't like them. If you have kids, you'll know they say they don't like something but have never tried those Brussel sprouts. Tastes do change, as you grow older.

Try new recipes and different ways of preparing the veggies. Just the way they are prepared can make a big difference. Try veggie soups and different salads. If your list of vegetables is small, eat them. However, don't let your dislike for a few veggies stop you from getting your weight off.

Excuse 10 - I Dislike Chopping Vegetables

Now we are getting fussy aren't we? If you are all by yourself, the vegetables aren't going to chop themselves. If married, you may enlist your spouse to help. Chopping vegetables is just symbolic of preparing the food. Maybe you don't like to cook. Yes, there may be more veggies in a weight loss diet, especially in salads and soups. There are many jobs we dislike doing in life, but they just need to be done.

There are ways around this. You can buy prepared food from some grocery stores. When we go to Gatlinburg Tennessee, we shop at a Food City, which has a salad bar. You can buy all the fixings for a salad and pay by the ounce. This salad can be a little more expensive than preparing from all the ingredients yourself but much more convenient. You don't have to buy all the fixings and waste what you don't use. This store also has hot food prepared. This is a tourist town and we tourists like convenience.

Most grocery stores have containers of chopped veggies in their produce section. They provide the convenience of just carrying home your veggies ready for soup, salad, or any other recipe. You pay other people to chop them, for the convenience.

There are also many devices, which make chopping fast and easy. They slice, shred, dice, and peel. Just slice dice and add some rice. Find ones, which clean up easy Charlene says.

There are always alternatives to excuses and this is just a weak excuse. Sometimes you need a swift kick or a little help thinking outside your preset boundaries. I once was a member of a diet message board who gave you a picture of a boot kicking someone's derriere when we made excuses such as this one. Turn on the TV and watch the news while you chop, or maybe find some chopping music, but don't make this excuse.

Excuse 11 - I Don't Like To Cook

Me neither. I'm fortunate I have a talented wife who does the cooking. So what happens if you don't cook or have a talented spouse to help? Sounds like a big problem for weight loss. I know some people just go out to eat and eating out is a real problem for the overweight.

If you really **can't** cook, then you can learn about cooking such as taking classes, watching Food Network, surfing the cooking websites, and joining cooking clubs. There are many YouTube videos to explain exactly what to do. There is no excuse for not knowing how to cook with so many ways available to learn the how's of cooking.

We are talking about someone who doesn't like to cook. You might not like the complicated recipes, so there are countless easy ones on the web. If you are cooking by yourself, maybe a class might bring some spark into your life. Meet others and see how they enjoy cooking.

Assuming you are not just lazy and you just really don't like to cook, there are more and more products available to help. You can find pre-cooked meats and veggies, frozen dinners matching your diet requirements. Just toss into the oven or microwave as directed for an easy meal. The "I Love This Diet" just uses frozen meals.

Many grocery stores have prepared foods. Choose wisely for good weight control. You can find pre-packaged salads ready to eat. You can eat well and not cook. Better yet, learn the fun in cooking and overcome the "I don't like to cook" excuse.

Excuse 12 - I Don't Like Fish

For me this is not an excuse but a fact. I can't stand the smell or the taste of fish. My mother doesn't and my daughter doesn't either. I'm definitely not like those people who love fish and the smellier the better.

Most diets use fish as a primary protein because fish is lower in fat and calories. Fish used to be cheap, but not anymore. When you flip back to Chapter 10 in a diet book and look for what you can eat, just remember there will always be some foods in a diet listing which you will not like. That's okay. I am not going to eat food I hate, just because it's on the diet or it's healthy. Most people like fish and fish fits their diet. I don't. I usually substitute chicken in place of fish.

Don't let anything on the diet keep you from dieting. For you it might not be fish but some other food. Charlene hated the smell of liver cooking when she was young. We are to enjoy food. It isn't just fuel.

Some varieties of fish I can eat, such as Albacore tuna in water, but they are not my favorite. I don't enjoy eating them. I tolerate them. Shrimp or lobster I like, but you might not classify them as fish. When you come across foods which you don't like, find a substitute or just omit them. I would never go on a seafood diet. I would rather go on a "see food" diet. I see it I eat it. Don't allow something listed on the diet be an excuse to not diet.

Excuse 13 - I Don't Like Water

Can you believe there are people who hate water when 60% of our body is water? We know most diets recommend drinking lots of water. The heavier you are the more water you should drink, and the more active you are the more water you should drink. Water has many health benefits as well as weight loss benefits. Water helps flush out the system and keeps the body hydrated and is mandatory for life.

I know you know all that stuff. You still hate to drink water. I want to say balderdash, but I know there are a few people who, for whatever reason, just hate to drink water. They have probably been drinking sodas and never water, so water tastes bland or tasteless. Water has no taste or at least shouldn't. Avoid stinky water. Use of water in cooking doesn't change the taste of the food as God designed water should be. I know in many places tap water doesn't taste so good. We spend quite a bit of time at the beach, and in most places, the water tastes like what I call beachy. We always go and buy bottled water at some of our destinations— Hilton Head comes to mind. You might need a filter. We have a whole house filter.

For some people it's not so much they hate water, as they don't like water. They'd drink water if they had to. There are ways to help. Put in some fruit, such as lemon, lime, strawberries, etc. I've even seen where people put in spices. I could take maybe cinnamon, cloves, ginger, or something similar. In fact, we had water with sliced cucumbers, mint, lemons, and grated ginger. It was good with meals.

There are many flavored waters available. Check the label of commercial flavored water. Some add sugar, sodium, or sweeteners. Some add vitamins. There are new products coming out each day, which might delight your taste buds and still get in the needed water. There are also some products for putting in water, but again watch the labels. Maybe just get use to drinking good old H$_2$O.

Excuse 14 - I Don't Want To Keep Track of Calories

The excuses we are talking about are excuses keeping you from a weight loss diet. The fact you don't like to keep track of your calories shouldn't keep you from a successful weight loss journey. I've done calorie tracking and I find it tedious. Trying to figure out how many calories are in a meal is hard. Food databases are getting very good and include many restaurant foods. However, it still comes up short unless you never eat out and you never fix a combined ingredient meal such as stew.

I believe those who keep track of calories in some way will do better than those who don't. Many diets will have lists of ingredients with amounts such as 1-cup cauliflower and have the meals already calculated. In fact, many diets have the calories already figured into them. One famous diet uses points instead of calories. They have already figured the calories out in the plan.

I also know after tracking food for a while you will get to know how many calories are in certain foods. If you restrict eating portions, you will also cut the calories. Many diets suggest you keep a diary for a while just to record all the food you eat. I read a blog where a person has done this throughout her weight loss journey and even her maintenance. If you aren't losing, then you can check the calories. You are probably eating too many. Calories are sneaky. Also, just fix your allowed food for each meal and put your meal on the plate so you won't eat extra. Don't sit bowls of mashed potatoes on the table.

If the diet you selected requires you to count calories and you don't want to, or don't have time, don't count them, or change your diet. Just don't make this an excuse to losing you weight.

Excuse 15 – I'll Just Gain It All Back and More

You probably will. Some say as high as 95% of dieters who lose weight will gain it back. Others say there is no good research showing exactly how many will gain the weight back. Let's just say the majority of people will gain the weight back. There are many reasons for weight gain including. emotions, failing to stay on a plan, going back to old habits, and unresolved issues making you gain weight in the first place, just to mention a few.

The person, who says they will gain the weight back, will gain the weight back. There is no total commitment to getting the weight off and keeping it off. The same reason that got the weight off should still help you keep off the weight. If the reason is health, through thick and thin health will always be your reason. Many people fall into the yo-yo diet by losing weight, gaining the weight back, going on another diet, losing weight, and gaining the weight back. I've been there and that cycle is exasperating to say the least.

Don't go on a diet, if your mental state is I'll just gain the weight back. Why bother. You have to have a reason to lose weight, which will sustain you through all the difficult times, and help you maintain your weight when you have reached your goal. Don't go into a weight loss journey without the desire to remove the weight and maintain your svelte figure the rest of your life.

Excuse 16 - I Didn't Realize It Had So Many Calories

If you don't count calories, you may not know how many calories some foods have. I had a co-worker many years ago who went on a diet. He wasn't having any success losing weight. We asked what he ate each day. He was eating fruit and vegetables mostly. We finally got down to the actual food he was eating and since he loved avocados, he ate several a day. The average avocado has 322 calories. He didn't realize they had so many calories.

Many foods the average person might eat contain many calories. Fast foods are loaded with calories. For example, a Big Mac meal has approximately 1350 calories, probably a day's worth. Also, oils and nuts can add up fast. A handful of peanuts (about 39) for example, are 170 calories. What weight challenged person can eat only a little handful?

Many restaurants have the calories on the menus. It is government mandated for larger chain restaurants. Some items are shocking at the number of calories in a meal. Eating out presents serious calorie problems for the weight loss journey, and we won't even mention the "all you can eat" places where you might eat a few days' worth of calories in one sitting.

Desserts can be sugar laden, but calorie laden as well. Cupcakes, for example can be 300 to 600 calories each. Eat more than one and the calories tally up fast.

Get on a good diet plan and you will eliminate most of those high calorie foods. They will have set amounts of calories you can eat for men and women. Stick to fruits, vegetables. Eat clean. Watch the avocados and don't over eat fruit. Two to three servings a day is plenty. Add good portions of protein to each meal such as low-calorie meats including chicken or turkey. Maybe a small amount of steak once or twice a week. Check the package label if it has one for the calories and you'll get a good idea the amount of calories *per* serving. Watch the serving size because chances are the package is more than one serving.

Learn about calories and their effect on dieting. Know the high calorie ones and avoid them. You need to be informed.

Excuse 17 – Looking Thin is Just Vanity

I'm not sure who would say this but somebody did. I think if I had a choice of looking thin or looking fat, I'd chose thin. I don't mean starvation thin. I realize that the media portrays the pretty people as thin and making that the standard for all pretty people is wrong. This is especially true for the younger age group.

Vanity is "excessive pride in or admiration of one's own appearance or achievements." Excessive pride is never good.

While I was writing this, I got an email that said, "Do you want to be beautiful and attractive with natural magnetic eyelashes?" The media and advertising pushes external beauty even if enhanced with artificial eyelashes. Now that might be vanity.

Everyone should like himself or herself as they are, in terms of happiness, contentment, and knowing God loves them just the way they are. However, for health reasons being overweight isn't good and really doesn't look good. I don't think it's vanity to want to see the excess weight gone in your life. Depending on your definition of thin, I think being at a God designed weight enhances you physically, and changes your view of yourself.

Excuse 18 - Diets Are Too Restrictive

Restrictive is a relative thought. Some people like strict guidelines to follow. Many people do not. Many diets fail because of the restrictions. The whole idea of constraints led many diet makers to attempt to answer the dilemma in some way.

One diet I'm thinking of in particular, has gotten around the restrictions by saying you can eat anything you want, but only when your body signals you are hungry, and you stop eating when your body signals you are full. Some say eating slowly gives your body a chance to signal when full, usually up to 20 minutes. However, we weight challenged folks aren't good about following body signals. We usually have our food eaten far before receiving any full signals. We keep eating even when we should have gotten the full signal. I remember as a growing youth, I'd eat dinner, get up from the table, and fix a sandwich.

Some diets try to give you the allusion it isn't restrictive by your eating large quantities of low-calorie foods such as lettuce. You think, wow I can't eat all this food. Some just cut one ingredient such as sugar or wheat. However, like eating Chinese food, you're hungry again in an hour. The "all you can eat" diets just say you can have this piece of pizza, and one slice is "all you can eat."

Weight loss diets are by definition somewhat restrictive. You have to cut the calories by 25% or so in order to create a calorie deficit. So yes, some diets such as the cabbage diet are very restrictive. All weight loss diets have the common goal of helping you get extra weight off your anatomy. I don't recommend eating cabbage soup each meal, but find a diet giving you enough food to keep from feeling you're getting nothing to eat.

Excuse 19 – I like Being Fat

I can't imagine anyone would say this, but some people do. One person said, "I'm a fat chick and love it." She also said she has 99 problems but being fat isn't one of them. Kids often bullied her because of her weight all through school and she hated herself for being overweight, however, she came to love who she was. Obviously, this is not a candidate for weight loss.

She is only 22 and still feels healthy, but statistics say it won't last. I'm the first to say you should be happy and confident in yourself totally apart from your size. Although she makes a living being a plus size consultant, she has not so great days ahead of her. I don't wish her any ill or any like her who like being fat, but I know God did not design the body to carry a bunch of extra weight. My counsel would be love yourself and begin to think about starting a weight loss journey, even if just small steps without becoming obsessive. If she thinks, she feels fine today, how would she feel if she didn't have to carry around a 100-pound knapsack all day?

Excuse 20 - All I Can Eat Is Sticks and Twigs

Wow, that is a strict diet. Sounds more like an animal diet than a people diet. This excuse is a metaphor for not getting those foods you ate which got you fat. I used to say sticks and twigs when I had a mixed green salad. Some of those lettuce varieties look like sticks and twigs, at least like weeds.

I think this is the myth of weight loss dieting. You don't get to eat much of anything good. How about if it tastes good, spit it out. You see the joke on sitcoms when one of the characters is dieting. They get a little carrot stick on their plate, when everyone else is eating lasagna. A good healthy weight loss diet is going to have gobs of veggies in the food list.

Vegetables are low in calories and provide good food for a weight loss diet. They are high in water content, and are nutritious and most are delicious. A good diet plan will have plenty of vegetables, but plenty of other foods also. I often have a plate consisting of a nice portion of chicken, veggies, and brown rice—no sticks and twigs. Dieting is not starving, or living on carrots or celery. There are wide varieties of foods meeting the diet recommendations, and you can fix them in countless ways making any diet delicious and interesting.

Yes, a few carrot and celery sticks are a fine snack.

Excuse 21 - I Don't Want To Starve Everyday

I don't want to either. The hardest part of a weight loss diet is feeling hungry. We have all seen the cartoon where a skeleton is sitting on the park bench which the caption, "He was on a diet." There is even a diet called the "No Hunger Diet." Such diets usually means lots of protein and fiber helping keep the belly fuller. With three meals and three snacks, you'd think you would never get hungry. The only diet you will literally feel starved on is the starvation diet. Yep, unbelievably, there are even starvation diets. I wouldn't recommend any of those. You will not starve on any normal weight loss diet. With 1200 to 1400 calories a day, your body will not go into starvation mode.

Most dieters will say they are starving when they get a few hunger pangs. The high schooler coming into the house after school will say he's starving. You may even fast a few days and your body will not starve. I know some people who have gone on a 40-day fast. I don't know if the fast was a water-only fast or liquid. Hey, you can liquefy a steak. Jesus went on a 40-day fast. Without any food, you will survive 30-40 days, maybe longer if you have a supply of fat reserved. Overall, starving isn't good.

Will you feel hungry at times—yes? Do you feel like you could eat more—yes? In order to lose weight, you have to eat less than your body wants, thereby forcing the body to go to the reserves—stored fat. Eating less can sometimes cause you to feel a bit hungry. Your body gets use to you feeding it. When you cut back, it tends to rebel. However, hunger is a long ways from starving. Charlene always says when your tummy growls, your body is chomping up the fat. Dieting does not mean starving, by a long shot. No excuses.

Excuse 22 – I'll Look Like a Chicken

Isn't that better than looking like a turkey or a pig? It's a myth to say you will get so skinny you'll have chicken legs. No one is saying you should get so small and thin. If you think so, then you need counseling, seriously. If you are already too thin, you need to go on a weight gain program. Of course, you aren't reading this book either.

Many of the excuses have to do with looks. However, who is considered healthy, the fat person or the thin? Whom do people consider fit, the fat, or the thin? Who are profiled as lazy, the fat or the thin. This society is thin conscious and they reward the thin.

I know it's superficial nonsense but the basis is looking healthy. Maybe you're self-consciousness thinking people are judging you, and if they are, too bad for them. This is you and your life. If you go on a weight loss diet, you aren't going to set a goal that makes you look like a chicken. Losing weight is difficult at best and you aren't going to lose more than you have to.

Excuse 23 - Do I have To Eat Organic?

Many diets call for organic food. Organic foods have been grown or farmed without the use of artificial chemicals, hormones, antibiotics, or genetically modified organisms (GMOs). Organic is also free of artificial food additives, artificial sweeteners, preservatives, coloring, flavoring, and monosodium glutamate (MSG). Organically grown crops usually use natural fertilizers and animals raised organically don't receive antibiotics or hormones.

Several studies have found organic foods generally contain higher levels of antioxidants and certain micronutrients, such as vitamin C, zinc, and iron. A review of 233 studies found a lack of strong evidence to conclude organic foods are more nutritious than regular foods. There is not enough strong evidence available to prove eating organic provides health benefits over eating regular foods.

So do you have to eat organic? Ange Alex, Holistic Health Practitioner, says eating organic can help remove the toxins in the system and keep them out. She would probably say yes, you get to eat organic as a healthy option. Do you have to eat organic? Of course you don't. Diets are not dictators, just guidelines. Should you eat organic, when the budget allows, probably. Work organic into your diet if you can. Wash your veggies with a veggie wash. Some veggies you can wash toxins from pesticides better than others do. Don't worry about it if you can't or just don't want to eat organic. We eat very little organic food.

Excuse 24 – As Long As I'm Healthy I'm not Worrying about My Weight

You shouldn't worry anyway because worrying is not healthy in itself. First, as St. John said, "Beloved, I wish above all things that thou mayest prosper and be in health, even as thy soul prospereth" (3 John 1:2). I hope you are healthy as long as you are here on the earth. In addition, I'm with you; I'm not going to worry about weight.

There are countless ways, which the body can get unhealthy. Smoking for example, is a definite risk to becoming unhealthy. Being overweight is certainly a risk to health. I'm for minimizing health risks wherever possible and practical. My father had two sisters. He and one sister were always thin. The other sister was plump. She outlived both of her thin siblings. So being a little heavy is not a sure sign you will be unhealthy.

However, God didn't design the body to carry extra weight. Joints begin to break down, and other diseases are more prevalent among the obese, such as diabetes. Most doctors will recommend you lose weight if you're overweight because they have seen the detrimental consequences of being overweight. Lose the weight and you'll just eliminate one potential health problem.

Excuse 25 - I Don't Get To Eat Out

If you are overweight, chances are you love to eat. Going out to restaurants and eating is one of your favorite pastimes. I fall into such a category. Eating out is both fun and entertaining, and a break from cooking. Some people just cannot give up eating all-you-can-eat pasta or all-you-can-eat pancakes at IHOP. Some places have great sandwiches I would have a hard time fixing at home. Eating out is great, but filled with minefields for the weight loss dieter.

I love to eat out, but restaurant food is often calorie expensive as well as financially expensive. One meal might cost you a day's worth of calories.

Do you have to give up eating out completely? Some diets restrict you from eating out for the first couple of weeks. However, you can eat out but you have to make wise and educated choices. Planning is the key. Know your eating plan and fit the restaurant menu into your plan.

I just don't go to some restaurants because they are too dangerous for my diet. Buffets and smorgasbords are very hazardous to my diet. Mexican and Italian are very difficult. If we are on a trip, we will often go online and check the menu. If we can find an item on their menu we can eat, then we go. If not, we cross the place off the list. While on a weight loss diet, you very well might have to limit your going out to eat. You can't make eating out an excuse.

Excuse 26 - They Have a Bogo

Buy 1 get one free. Some grocery stores heavily push Bogos. I just looked at an ad from one of these stores and the Bogos are for foods such as soda, chips, ice cream, pasta, mayonnaise, cookies, crackers, and cereal—all the groceries the average weight loss diet doesn't include. They had a couple of items on usual diets, such as organic tomatoes, frozen vegetables, humus, and spring water.

Bogos are a good deal—50% off and are hard to pass up. In fact, you should take advantage of any discounts you can find, unless you have too much money. You just have to make sure you don't fall for unhealthy choices. Some stores have other types of discounts. Twofer, multiples for a discounted price such as 10 for $10, and weekly loss leaders to get you into the store. Use all these tools to get your food budget down. You can sometimes find clearance items on a special shelf. Just don't take the donuts.

Pick and choose wisely the products fitting your diet. Don't just buy a bag of chips because they are buy one get one FREE. Free doesn't mean it's good for your weight loss journey.

Excuse 27 – I Get Bonus Points

Okay, you got me on there. Companies give you bonus points in an attempt to keep you coming. Many will give you something free if you buy five. One gas station for example gives you free coffee each month when you reach a certain level. Many fast food companies have similar bonus plans.

I'm a Starbucks fan. They offer bonus stars as rewards for spending there. Reach 125 points and you get a free drink of your choice. They also have double point days, and happy hours Bogos. I usually have several free drinks available when I go on trips and use them then. Challenges for something free are addicting. The game companies always have some challenge going on all the time to keep you involved—and spending. Some places have games to get you in multiple times a day, during weekends, and during the slower afternoon hours.

If you like the challenge then okay as long as the contest doesn't interfere with your weight loss plan. However, you have to use a little wisdom and not overdue it especially if it involves food. If you need to buy five hamburgers to get one free, you might not be making the correct weight loss decision. Low calories and healthy is the plan of most diets, and most diets don't recommend fast food.

Excuse 28 - But It's Free

"But it's free," or as in the case of buffets, the more you eat the less your meal costs per item. This free food shows up now and then when you are dieting. We all like free. I always look at the free samples at Trader Joe's when we go. There is a Peanut Shop in Williamsburg, VA that puts out free samples. Fudge shops are always luring you in with the promise of free samples. Conferences and work meetings have their share of free food around.

The last time we went to the resort in St. Augustine, they were giving out free M&M's celebrating Father's Day. They also hand out candy during Halloween and there are some resorts we visit which hand out free cookies. My dad was very frugal and always joked his ancestors were Scottish. I'm thinking he heard the word scotch, meaning cheap and tied it to Scotland. I don't think that is true, but being frugal is not bad. I picked up the frugal gene so I love free stuff.

However, free when dieting could come with hidden costs. Your progress will slow down and even temporarily stall your weight loss journey. In addition, as I have found more often than not, I'm on the edge of a slippery slope to getting off track. If you eat a food not on plan, you have to compensate for the extra calories. So beware of free and stick to the plan.

Excuse 29 – It's 50% Off!

Some time ago, I had to pick up a particular item at a big store. I zoomed in, heading for the aisle I needed. As I approached an aisle facing me on the left, I saw many people standing around gazing at the items on the shelves. Even a store employee led someone to the area as well. All the activity got my attention so I turned to see *what* was so special about the items on *those* shelves. CANDY. They had stacked the leftover Easter candy on those shelves. What wasn't surprising was each shelf displayed a **50% OFF** sign.

I can appreciate a good sale, but I continued walking while processing what I'd seen. Then I noticed something sad. The majority of people gawking and pawing at the 50% off candy were very *overweight*. I understand their excitement because they're saving money, but I also thought how sad. Just because an item is 50% OFF doesn't mean it's a good healthy choice for you. Don't fall for the hype especially if the edibles are not on your weight loss plan.

Go for the good, healthy foods instead. Maybe you'll find some 50% off sales over there.

Excuse 30 – I'll Look Older If I lose Weight

I've seen that problem. However, I am old. When I am a little overweight, my face fills in and you don't see the wrinkles so much. When I lose the weight, my skin sags and I get chicken neck. Have you seen heavy people and then next time you see them they are thin. Their thinness almost scares you. Yet they look so much better.

Experts say losing weight slowly is better than losing quickly, because you lose more muscle, which helps support the skin tissues. Therefore, be sure and hydrate well. In addition, you need plenty of exercise, which will strengthen and tighten your skin.

Face exercises are a little more of a problem. You might consider some supplements that help such as collagen which you can take in powder or pill form.

Some doctors say that saggy skin will go away eventually as the skin begins to reshape itself. So far, I haven't seen that affect much. If you lose a lot of weight, then you might need some cosmetic surgery for saggy skin. Some people Botox the wrinkles. I'm not sure medical procedures are worth it, but I'm not judging those who do.

Again, we are talking about looks. Why do we focus so much on looks? Who is deciding if we look good or not? What is the standard? The Cosmetic industry is a multibillion-dollar enterprise. I try to look my best according to my standard. However, if I lose the weight that could be making me unhealthy and I get a little sagging skin because of the loss, so be it.

Excuse 31 - I Paid For It

I paid for it so I don't want to waste it. My first thought to this excuse was, if you don't "waste" it, you will "waist" it. I grew up in a family where there wasn't any extra money and my dad was shall we say, frugal. I saw him eat a meal, and obviously was full, but kept eating because he was not going to waste food.

How many parents use the ruse you have to eat everything on your plate because there are starving children in China? I could never understand the thinking in the statement. How did cleaning my plate help the starving children in China? Sending my plate of food to them would help more. I know it was really saying we should be grateful for the food we have because others aren't so fortunate.

Approximately 40 percent of food in the U.S. goes to waste, meaning roughly one-third of the food produced in the world for human consumption every year—approximately 1.3 billion tons— is lost or wasted. Wasted food is such a waste when there are people who need food. I don't like waste.

Plan your meals so there isn't any waste. Don't buy food you shouldn't eat. Plan your grocery shopping so everything is used. Buy only food on your plan in the quantities needed. Don't pay for extra, so you don't have to waste anything. Unless you have several in your family, the stores that sell in bulk might not be a place you should go, unless you really plan carefully.

Excuse 32 - All I Drink Is Coffee

This excuse was probably in response to the question, "What do you drink on the diet?" There is always a debate as to whether coffee or tea counts as water. Women require about 90 ounces (11 cups) of fluids per day, while men should aim to get around 125 ounces (16 cups) per day. Even the tried and true eight glasses a day is good. What about the coffee and tea controversy? Can you count them as water? You make coffee and tea from water so I count it as water. Many used to believe coffee was dehydrating, but the myth has been debunked. The diuretic effect does not offset hydration. The problem is caffeine. Some of us have to watch carefully our intake of caffeine. Too much and my heart starts making extra beats.

People usually drink coffee for the energy boast especially in the mornings. Some people especially young people are drinking caffeine boasted drinks. I personally don't recommend them.

I go to Starbucks almost every day. There are many more varieties of "coffee" drinks. I get the skinny mocha with almond milk. It's low in calories and Charlene and I usually share a small one or more correctly a tall one.

When people say they only drink coffee, I always ask what they put in the coffee. Some fill the cup half full of cream and sugar. I watched one person put 7 teaspoons of sugar in his coffee. Sugar isn't on anyone's weight loss plan. Too much coffee can throw off a weight loss plan, and some diets limit coffee.

If you drink more than two cups of coffee a day, you are probably addicted to coffee. Stop drinking it for a few days and see what the withdrawal symptoms are like—headaches. If all you drink is coffee, then start drinking more water. I drink decaf when I do drink coffee. I don't get the pick-me-up you get from regular coffee, but you get the taste and the relaxing moment in the morning. However, you can still do a weight loss program whether you drink coffee or not.

Excuse 33 - I Can't Stand the Cravings

There are two types of cravings—real and imagined. Real cravings come from a diet deficient in something your body needs to keep itself healthy. Your body could be low or deficient in certain micronutrients—vitamins, minerals, and antioxidants. Some diets restrict certain macronutrients such as carbs, fat, or protein. Your body has a warning mechanism telling you to replace needed supplies. You may need to adjust your diet.

Speaking of cravings, I'll bet you get them all the time whether you are on a weight loss diet or not. The difference is you give into the cravings more easily and run to the vending machine and get a candy bar or a bag of potato chips. While on a diet, you have to put aside those cravings or deal with them someway instead of running to the vending machine.

If the cravings aren't real, then those imagined cravings are a completely different story. You had your usual snack cake in the evening for 20 years. You go on a diet, and Little Debbie snack cake is not on the plan. The first night on the diet, you're craving your Ding Dong—emotional craving. Life seems somehow "normal" when you have your Ding Dong.

Your mind thinks you are supposed to have a snack. Your body could be experiencing any number of cravings, all emotional attachment to food. The day was crazy, but is back to normal when you have your usual snack. Those cravings are going to take some work to overcome. You have to learn to say no. You may be able to find an alternate on your plan, maybe a few grapes or a few apple slices. Mental cravings can be tough, but you can overcome even this excuse.

Excuse 34 - I Can't Curb My Cravings

Much like the previous excuse, this one is about cravings. This one also uses the awful word "can't." To me "can't," says it is impossible, but we all know nothing is impossible. A food craving is an intense desire to consume a specific food, and is different from normal hunger. You will experience cravings on a diet just as you experience them while not on a diet.

People often crave foods with high levels of sugar glucose, such as chocolate, than foods with lower sugar glucose, such as broccoli. This is because when glucose interacts with the opioid receptor system in the brain it triggers a desire for more. Carbs, such as crackers or potato chips are also a source of craving, especially if salted. Cravings are very common. In fact, more than 50% of people experience cravings on a regular basis and weight loss diets can cause more craving.

Take cravings as a challenge to overcome. Have a plan that reduces cravings. Eat plenty of protein. Drink lots of water. Eat fruit, which will help satisfy the sweet craving. Many hankerings come from a lack of something your body needs. Take a multi-vitamin to get needed vitamins and minerals. Reduce stress. Avoid places causing craving, such as don't hang out in the food court or the bakery. Know your triggers and avoid them.

Depending on the craving, you may be okay to give into it. If it is a chocolate craving, then you can figure a small piece of chocolate into your diet plan. One person lost over one hundred pounds and still had a small piece of chocolate every day, not easy for some.

Cravings will come but you can overcome with planning and by taking control of them.

<u>Excuse 35 - I Hate to Watch What I Eat</u>

I first thought this meant you didn't like to watch yourself eating. Maybe you were sitting in front of a mirror while you ate. However, I know you meant you don't want to have to choose diet food but would rather just eat what you want, the definition of not being on a diet.

Hate is a strong word, which will derail any attempt to lose weight. I would say if this is your excuse, you are not much of a candidate for weight loss. None of us likes to have to choose one food over another in order to lose weight. Let's see, a piece of chocolate cake or an apple. Us weight challenged folk will choose the chocolate cake every time.

So we need a really good reason to lose weight. A reason, which will override our dislike, to have to choose "diet food." There is also the whole idea of changing your likes to include food, which enhances your weight loss efforts. Make up your mind to eat on plan, lose the weight, and love how you look.

<u>Excuse 36 - No Healthy Place to Eat Near Work</u>

I'm assuming you work and you want to go out for lunch. Remember, we give an excuse to avoid going on a weight loss journey. So you came up with this one. You might think there is no healthy place, but in my experience, you can get items on your plan most anywhere. You may not find an organic health food café nearby, but you can find a diet friendly item on most menus.

When I was working, our team would go out for pizza occasionally. I love pizza, but overeating pizza will put on weight. You just have to use portion control. I know for a weight challenged person, portion control requires a great deal of restraint and discipline and might be in short supply. Try eating one piece of pizza.

There are going to be times when eating out for lunch will present problems. Instead of excuses, we want solutions. The meal has to fit into your plan or you may have to adjust your plan for the day. A piece or two of pizza for lunch may mean a small salad for dinner and doing some extra walking.

If you are eating lunch out with friends, okay. Pick an item you can eat. Salads are a good option. I know going out to lunch with friends or coworkers is a social occasion, but staying on the straight and narrow plan is also important. Going off plan for one meal can delay any loss for the week.

I would think about staying in and taking lunch to work that fits within your plan. I used to take my cooler to work with what I needed to eat for the day. Then do some walking during lunchtime. I've enjoyed many lunch times in the lunchroom getting to know people and saving the cost of going out. Don't use this excuse to keep you from your weight loss destiny.

Excuse 37 - What about My Mocha?

I'm a Starbucks fan. I've gotten countless rewards for drinking my mocha. Actually, in my defense drinking a skinny mocha. Therefore, this is my often-used excuse. I'm using mocha as my favorite food I don't want to give up while on a diet. For you the food could be something else.

So how do I get around this? Well, I put it on my plan. My diet allows me 8 ounces of milk a day, about 90 calories. A Venti mocha with whole milk and whipped cream is 490 calories. A tall is 310 calories, with non-fat milk, 250 calories, and without whipped cream, 190 calories. Buy a 110-calorie skinny mocha and use Almond milk and the total is 80 calories. I split the cup with my wife and now only 40 calories, only half my milk allowance.

You see where I'm going with this. There are often alternatives to your favorite. Even 110 calories split is only 55 calories. I still get my mocha and my plan is happy. Therefore, I turned my excuse into a workable solution, which fits my weight loss plan. Works for me and I no longer have an excuse shackling my chances of losing weight.

Whatever it is you don't want to give up, find a way to incorporate into you plan. If it's a six-pack, then forget it. Even one regular soda may be one too many. There will be times on the journey we will have to sacrifice certain foods we think we can't do without, but we really can.

Excuse 38 - I Have to Have My Evening Ice Cream

This is similar to the previous excuse, but expanded to those dangerous evenings in front of the TV. I realize there are people who think they must have their evening snack regardless. I've known people who eat ice cream every evening. The snack becomes a friend and comforts them from the daily stresses. The diet I was on gave me some pudding every evening and I got used to it and wanted it every evening.

Now if the snack fits into your plan, okay, but eating a bowl of ice cream, maybe not. Ben & Jerry's chocolate chip cookie dough ice cream is 270 calories for only ½-cup serving. I know from being an experienced ice cream eater ½ a cup isn't going to do it. Therefore, if we said 1 cup for 540 calories, then 1/3 of our daily calories will go to one snack. Not going to make the plan.

So first, you don't **have** to have your ice cream. Plainly said, you **want** your ice cream. You are not committed to the weight loss process. If you want your ice cream, then you want to be fat. If you are overweight, then just a taste won't work either. Weight loss does mean some changes in thinking.

Therefore, we find a way to have our cake and eat it too. In this case, our ice cream. There are many low calorie "ice creams" for less than 300 calories per pint. There are ice cream bars for less than 200 calories and some from 70 to 100 calories. There are alternates like nonfat yogurt and sugar free puddings. Where there is a will there is a way and ice cream too.

Excuse 39 - Bread And Butter Comes With the Meal

On special occasions, we go to O'Charley's restaurant and their first matter of business is to bring out their yeast rolls and butter. Now most diets won't have these on their plans. However, they come with the meal. I didn't grow up during the Great Depression, but my parents did. My Dad was particularly frugal. We ate out very seldom but if the server offered him "free" bread, he would have his share. He would always order chopped steak, which my Mom said he liked, but was the cheapest item on the menu. Coincidence? I don't think so.

I remember one restaurant had French bread, and we warned the waiter we liked lots of bread. After making three trips with the three pieces per table rule, he got mad and brought us a full and overflowing basket of delicious French bread. We ate it all. After all, it was "free."

We have on occasion told the server at O'Charley's not to bring out any bread. I think I'm a little like my dad and telling the server to not bring out bread brings tears to my eyes. Eating only one roll is also hard. The dieting correct thing to do is tell them "no bread," because you don't need the added calories. On Wednesday, they have free pie day. I find it interesting seeing the place is packed and people are waiting in line on free pie Wednesdays. I guess it's not surprising people flock to "free." The same on "all you can eat" meals as well. All you can eat catfish and there's a line around the block. This is one excuse hard to do away with, but we need to eliminate from our diet vocabulary and practice. We have to watch out for the free stuff. Extra calories make the weight loss journey difficult. Notice I said "We."

Excuse 40 - I Won't Give Up My Soda

Soda is symbolic of all the sugary drinks available. Whether Soda, pop, soda pop, fizzy, carbonated soft drink, even coke when it's not, all falls under this excuse. Many people have some drink they just don't want to give up. As an example, let's look at Coke for this excuse. A 12 oz. can is 140 calories with 39 grams of sugar. Most people who won't give up soda drink more than one a day, in fact, several a day. You can see this soda pop is going to keep making you fat and unhealthy if you refuse to give it up. Sugary drinks won't fit in any diet. This excuse is, "I would rather be fat than give up my soda." A diet version has one calorie. Would you be willing to switch to diet even though experts will say diet drinks are still not healthy? Besides, most caffeine-laden drinks **are addictive.**

Health apparently isn't a concern for this person. We are talking now about fitting this into a diet. I know a person who won't give up Coke Zero. He has several a day. Though there are no calories, there is plenty of caffeine, artificial sweeteners, caramel coloring, i.e., not too healthy and possibly inflammatory. Everyone has the choice to make. Some foods will just not fit a healthy weight loss lifestyle. You have to choose what you want most. Health is precious and making it a priority seems a sensible way to go. There are foods on a weight loss diet you just have to give up or you aren't on a weight loss diet.

Excuse 41 - People Always Bring Food to Work

When I was working, there was food in the break room almost every morning. Some people were just nice and fixed a plate full to bring in, while others were simply getting rid of extra food. Either way, I always got my coffee when there was a chance something else would be there. The day after Halloween there was bowls of candy. One of my coworkers often brought in donuts. All this "free" food is hard to pass up. This breakroom food was all helpful in making me obese. The best idea would have been to avoid the break room in the morning. I could have waited until 10:00 and got my coffee. I could have just ignored the food. Yeah right...that didn't work.

However, as you know, giving up free food is difficult for weight challenged people to do. I know some people who never went to the break room, even when someone announced over the loudspeaker there was pizza in the break room. When I heard the announcement, I ran, well, walked very fast. Pizza doesn't last long in a break room nor does a cake, donuts, or sweets.

You can't stop people from bringing food and stuff. You have to deal with it. The best way of course is to flee. Just don't go to where food might be located. It's easier not to go near the snacks, than to refrain from taking some once you see them. Just another challenge the weight loss dieter has to overcome, if he or she wants to make progress.

This reminds me of one particular challenge a major TV reality program gave to those wanting to lose weight. They could gain immunity for the next week and be guaranteed to stay another week IF they did not give in to eating anything in the test room. One by one, the contestants entered. Some gawked at all the food. Some just stood and smelled in the delicious aromas. Others ignored the discipline of walking away and ate what they could. Some calculated how many calories they were eating and would stop when they reached a certain number. Again, the best course of action is just to flee, leave the room and don't look back.

Excuse 42 - I Need My Chocolate

I was reading an article about women who had lost more than 100 pounds and how they did it. Here's a quote. "One or two dark chocolate peanut butter cups. I have dark chocolate almost every day—I love it and it helps me avoid feeling deprived or restricted." This woman still lost although she had her chocolate. My wife and I like chocolate semi sweet chips. We have a few after a meal. I guess what I'm saying is a diet doesn't have to be so strict you can't enjoy anything special.

You just have to be careful to figure it into you daily calorie allotment. 1 oz. of dark chocolate has 170 calories, 14% of a 1200 calories allotment. Learn to replace it with other items such as fruit. Have your chocolate for special treats occasionally. The problem I have and maybe many dieters have is they can't stop at 1 oz. We tried that with a bar, breaking off one square at a time. However, the bar was soon gone. God's grace says everything is legal to eat, but not everything is profitable to your weight loss journey.

Chocolate is just an example of a treat you might really want while on your diet. Maybe it's a cookie, or I know one person who has some yogurt every evening. Just fit it into the plan.

Excuse 43 - I Always Get a Diet Soda

Have you ever bought a Big Mac, large fries, an apple pie, and then a diet soda? I have to laugh because I've done that—often. Well, at least you are not getting the sugar. A typical drink at a fast food restaurant is a 16 oz. coke, and weighs in at 192 calories and contains 51 grams of sugar. A diet version has 16 calories and 1 gram of sugar. So choosing diet is better than a regular soda. We aren't looking at the healthiness of any of these products here, but the point being you can't overeat in one area and hope to lose by eating less in another area.

To me diet soda tastes better than regular coke. If you have been dieting for long you won't like food so sweet. I remember loving to bite into a Krispy Kreme donut. They just melt in your mouth. I hadn't bought any for years until a Krispy Kreme store opened near us. I went during St. Patrick's week and the donuts were green. I bought some and bit into the donut waiting for the delicious melt in my mouth, and the donut was so sweet I could hardly eat it, though I did anyway.

I usually get water with my meals and on occasion unsweetened ice tea. Even then, by overeating and then thinking by drinking water you're doing well is a partial lie. You are doing good drinking water, but not well on how much you eat.

I think a person could eat whatever they wanted if they ate in the right portions—moderation experts say. The number of calories a day is what counts. One slice of pizza would fit into a meal plan. A healthy piece of pizza even better. So don't try to kid yourself into thinking you are doing well on your diet by drinking a diet soda while eating 1200 calories. No excuses.

Excuse 44 – It's Evening In Front Of the TV

You might have the problem of sitting for several hours in front of the TV in the evenings. Actually, spending time in front of the TV could happen anytime of day. I think this is my excuse—or one of them.

If you sit in front of the TV for any length of time in the evening, eventually you will want to snack. You will endure several food commercials and they just subliminally reach into your brain and rattle a snack out of you. I think watching food commercials require a tremendous effort of will to ignore the urge to eat something. The alternative is to have a snack on your plan you can eat, such as fruit, nuts, veggies rather than crackers, cookies, and candy.

I don't like to drink liquid later as I then have to get up in the middle of the night for a bathroom trip. Several fruits work great such as an apple, strawberries, blueberries, pears, melons, and oranges. We sometimes enjoy half of a baked apple or homemade applesauce.

You want to have a diet plan that includes the evening snack if no evening snack is troublesome. The more restrictions you place on yourself the harder the diet will be. Therefore, where you have weaknesses such as evening time, try to find low-calorie, healthy snacks giving you a physical and emotional boast. Don't run to McDonald's when you see their Big Mac ad.

Excuse 45 - The Expiration Was Tomorrow

Now some of us hate to waste food. We would rather eat it since we paid for it. What do you mean expiration date? For us consumers, you will find normal food with a sell-by date on perishables like meat, seafood, poultry, and milk. The date is a guide for stores to know how long they can display a particular product. For the most part the date is a guide for us as well as to how fresh the product is. These dates are established guidelines and the products will last longer when you take them home, but not much longer. Most stores keep up on those dates and remove the product. The other date is "use by" or "best if used by" and you will generally find on shelf-stable products. This can easily last longer even years.

Enough said because this is just an excuse to eat. The ice cream says *best if used by tomorrow*, so you think you have a ready excuse to overeat. Why do you have ice cream? Not going to work.

Our son tends to let foods go too long many times. He doesn't like eating the same meal over again too soon so a half-opened package of something will sit in the fridge to the point you have to smell the product to see if it's any good. If in doubt, throw it out. Get the longer dates when you buy food. We always check the milk in the back because they put the closer dates to the front to sell them first. Sounds like a senior. Watch your food dates and plan ahead to use them before this becomes a problem and turns into an overeating excuse. If you have to throw it out do so, then you won't waist it.

Excuse 46 – It's Fat Free

I assume you aren't eating vegetables. When I write about these excuses, the excuse is just kicking the tires of the weight loss diet. The excuse is about eating an item not on your eating plan while on a weight loss diet.

The low-fat craze came out in the late 70's and strangely, obesity began to rise dramatically. This is when saturated fat became the villain and people began eating less red meat and more white meat. They also went from whole milk to skim. However, obesity climbed as well as other diseases. This was supposed to be the cure-all for heart disease. The medical community is still using the low-fat recommendations. The subject is complicated and controversial.

Therefore, fat-free isn't all it's claimed to be. In fact, fat-free may be hurting us rather than being a healthier choice. These products typically have labels saying, "low-fat" – "reduced fat" or "fat-free."

Replacing saturated fat with polyunsaturated fat such as olive oil may have health benefits such a reducing inflammation. The body needs a certain amount of fat to function properly and a no fat diet would be harmful. The problem with fats is they are high calorie. There are 9 calories per gram compared to 4 calories with carbs and protein.

The problem is food manufacturers replace fat with carbs such as sugar but they usually end up tasting like cardboard and they may hinder weight loss. No one would want to eat them. Research has shown sugar is worse than fat. So low fat is not the great excuse and in fact, may deter weight loss. If you are on a doctor prescribed low fat diet, follow your doctor's instructions. Also, in defense of low fat, there are low fat diets if they fit your emotional, mental, and physical needs.

Excuse 47 – It's A Family Tradition

I heard of a family who always meets at Golden Corral on Friday night for dinner. You are fortunate if your family lives nearby and you can get together. Now I'm all for family traditions. We have always had a family custom of going out to eat on any of our birthdays and allowing the birthday person to choose the place. My earliest remembrance of this was allowing our three-year-old daughter to choose her restaurant when we were in Kingston, New York on business. Of all the great-to-eat places such as Italian, she wanted KFC. We got KFC and ate chicken in our motel room. She was happy, and the budget was happy. Course, her tastes grew, and now no more KFC. Her family just came through on a RV trip and yes, we went out to eat for her birthday but not to KFC.

There is something about the family gathering together from time to time for a meal. Gathering around the table and enjoying a meal is a special time. Golden Corral gives everyone a chance to pick what they want, and overeat. Do you see a problem? An all you can eat place is never good for a dieter. A person with great will power could go to a buffet and eat, but the sight of so much food leads most overweight people astray. Buffets are why we are overweight.

Sadly, many overweight people have overweight families. My experience is one meal at an all you can eat place will set you back several days in your weight loss journey. If you have to go to maintain family unity, go and try your best to eat what's on your plan—start with a big salad and gobs of veggies, a small piece of meat, and skip the dessert bar—yipes.

Excuse 48 - It Was In the Fridge

Hey, if you find something in the fridge, it's fair game. If you are on a weight loss diet, you shouldn't be in the fridge unchaperoned, or in the kitchen for that matter according to my wife. In addition, every item in the fridge should be on plan. When I go look in the fridge for a snack, I'll only find veggies—no cheese or deli meats, etc. We don't normally cook more than a meal's worth so not a lot of leftovers are in our fridge. This excuse really involves other thinking, such as emotional eating, cravings, or simple sneak attacks.

Stay out of the fridge. Of course, I'm talking about unscheduled trips to the fridge. Take a step back and rethink your reason for opening the refrigerator. Then grab a glass of water and go back to what you were doing.

If you are not planning snacks into your diet, then you probably should. We have a mid-morning snack usually of fruit. We have a mid-afternoon snack and usually something in the evening. We like a baked apple with cinnamon. We might just have a sugar-free hot chocolate or some veggies. There are plenty of low calories snack options if you need them. Search the internet on that option and you will find yourself a snack. Stay out of the fridge.

Excuse 49 – What's For Lunch?

This doesn't sound like an excuse, however, when said can quickly lead to an excuse. I know because I say this often and it sometimes leads to going out to lunch. I'm not against people who own or work in restaurants and fast food places. Without someone going out to lunch, they wouldn't have income for daily necessities. However, for the overweight, going out to lunch is a challenge. Calories will be much higher than eating at home on plan.

The best idea is to stick to your plan. You do have a plan don't you. Getting use to sticking to the plan is difficult and going off the plan is easy. Therefore, learning to stay with the plan will help your weight loss process go better and help you reach your weight loss goal faster. So instead of asking what's for lunch, just look at your plan and fix your lunch. Don't think about hamburgers at your favorite place. Just stay the course and rejoice in your good decisions.

Excuse 50 - Just One Won't Hurt

Boy, how many times have I said that? This is a weight loss dieter's nightmare. Back in 1983, Lay's Potato Chips came out with the saying, "Betcha can't eat just one." This was in reference to their potato chips. Of course, you can't eat just one. Why would you go buy a bag, open the bag, and eat just one? Therefore, over the airwaves came the thinking most dieters had about food in general. No, we can't eat just one cookie. No, we can't eat just one slice of pizza. That's why we are overweight. Obesity begins with one—chip, cookie, donut, or whatever.

Yes, just one will hurt. I have found through many years of observation and experience eating something not on the diet will lead to a slippery slope of diet failure. You eat a few cookies and then you say well, I can be very good tomorrow. Some say the restriction is the problem. If you say you can't have cookies, then cookies are what you want most. So eat one they say. They don't know the dieter, as they should. The weight challenged are weight challenged because they can't eat just one.

I remember a minister shared his overeating bread experience. Although bread was his downfall, he won the battle by eliminating bread altogether, got his weight down, and was healthier than before.

A weight loss diet by definition means you have to avoid some foods causing you to be overweight. You have to develop a new mindset of thinking—as the Bible says, to renew your mind. Temptation of eating one will lead to another. So avoid the first one altogether.

Excuse 51 - I Have No Time for Breakfast

Some people think a proper diet always includes a healthy breakfast. Those people would be right. Breakfast means breaking the overnight fast. There is no shortage of expert opinions on how important breakfast is. That said then, we have to overcome the time problem. I'm assuming this means you are so busy with kids etc. you have no time. The kids eat, why not you? Do you need a course in time management? Would getting up 10 minutes earlier fix the problem? I hope this isn't a case of sleeping to the last minute and rushing out the door.

Maybe some planning would help. Prepare ahead for a quick breakfast. Do a search for meals you can prepare ahead. You don't need a whole three-course meal. Dieting is hard enough. Not eating breakfast will cause a hunger strike mid-morning. You can always take something for a snack to substitute for a skipped breakfast, but don't make skipping breakfast a habit. Don't put yourself in a position of being hungry and skipping breakfast will make you hungry. Work out the planning and taking care of yourself. Teach the kids to get their own cereal. Don't buy into this excuse.

Excuse 52 - I Love Fast Food

Did you know there are people out there in radio land who have never had a Big Mac? Do you know some of them did not eat a Big Mac on purpose? I have eaten Big Macs, and I ate them on purpose. I like fast food, and it is a potential problem for me. I guess we have to ask, what's wrong with fast food? I consider fast food as any place you have to stand at the counter to order your food. Fast food isn't necessarily bad, but often highly processed with large amounts of carbohydrates, added sugar, unhealthy fats, and salt (sodium). In addition, they use some gross ingredients to save money and prep time.

The draw for fast food is it is fast and rather cheap. You can grab a bag of food on your way home and feed the family food they love. I'm not going to rant and wail about fast food. Some places do have some healthy choices, but even then, beware. All chicken isn't created equal. Some fast food chains offer a healthier menu. Pollo Tropical, Chipotle, Pollo Loco, and the like serve delicious and what I would call healthier alternatives. Of course, the purist out there will always disagree.

The problem is calories for the weight loss dieter—high calories. Putting aside the health issues, calories are the culprit to weight loss failure. I know some people have gone on a fast food diet and lost weight, but eating fast food takes careful choices, and lots of walking or jogging to see weight loss. Until you get your weight off, bypass the fast food places and after goal only on rare occasions.

Excuse 53 - Fast Food Is Fast

Fast food is after all, fast. When you have a very limited amount of time, grabbing a quick bite at a fast food place is convenient. In the last excuse, we talked about fast food, but we didn't address the fact it is fast. Del Taco or Taco Bell can fix your 10 tacos before you can even fill up your cup of iced tea. All these fast food places feature drive-thru windows so you can get your food and be on your way. Our society is always in a hurry. Your 30-minute lunchtime is only 15 and you have to be at your next appointment.

At one place, I worked, I noticed the workers ate very fast and went out to play basketball during the rest of their lunch break. We live in the instant microwave society. We have instant pudding, instant oats, instant rice, instant soup, and of course, Ramen noodles. The family doesn't sit down together because they are all off doing something.

The fact they call it "fast food," indicates to me they sell the fact it is fast. People want fast, so sell them what they want. However, fast doesn't change the reality of being high calorie and contributes to the obesity epidemic today. Therefore, slow down or as the signs say Stay calm and eat slowly. Your weight loss will thank you.

Excuse 54 - Fast Food Is Cheap

Well, you got me there. Del Taco sells a taco for 69¢. Many places have $1 menus. Moreover, you don't have to prepare anything. The food is cheap for a reason. They are always looking for ways to cut costs, so something has to give, whether quality, quantity, or attempts to get a person to buy the more expensive food—"do you want to supersize that?" By the way, a 69¢ taco is small, and you'll end up eating at least five, but you can't beat the price.

I remember many years ago I was on a business trip and lived on per diem. I could get a hamburger, fries, and drink for about a dollar. I ate in the company cafeteria for cheap, so ended up saving money each week. A recent survey showed the average MacDonald's bill per person is \$4.72. My daughter has a family of five so that's \$23.60 for a meal and if Grandma and Grandpa come and pay the bill, it's \$33.04. Now not looking so cheap. Cost of pizza is even more. It might be convenient especially if you add prep time, but fast food still comes with a cost.

Excuse 55 - I End up Eating My Kid's Sweet Snacks.

I don't have this problem as I don't have kids around anymore. However, two problems stand out. First, why are you feeding your kids sweet unhealthy snacks? There are plenty of healthy snacks for kids and so change what they get use to eating. Changing their snacks can be difficult but not impossible; after all, you are the parent who supplies the food. Don't have unhealthy snacks in the house. Not surprising how a child will change his or her eating habits if only good foods are available.

Second, the choice is yours on what you eat. You can choose not to eat the kid's snacks if they don't fit your plan, but I suspect with a little planning their snacks could be your snacks. Stick to your plan. Have only the snacks on your plan if you buy snacks. I have found a snack helps the dieter make the journey from meal to meal easier.

You don't want your child to come home from school and ask where is my snack, and you have to say you ate them. Not good.

Excuse 56 – I'm The Only One Eating a Salad

In other words, I feel funny only eating a salad. This probably applies when going out to eat with co-workers, friends, or lunch after church. Wow, eating salads make you feel funny. A steak must make you totally giddy. I guess you are normally not funny.

Okay, I know this excuse means you are embarrassed or self-conscious about eating salads when everyone else is eating pizza or wings. If you are concerned about what people think then you need to get over it. Why do you care what everyone else thinks? You're the only one who is eating correctly. Your weight loss diet should be more important than what others might say. I know easier said than done.

First, if they say something cruel, they are not friends. Second, you're probably the only one even thinking about what you eat. Third, you might just have issues about what other people say about you. I grew up with self-conscious issues—always concerned about what others thought about me. Overcoming the issue is not easy. At some point, you just have to say, I'm me, and I don't care what others think about me. You have to be you. As Sammy Davis Jr, sang, "I gotta be me."

If you are on a weight loss diet, then your weight is more important than worrying about what others think about you going on a diet. You are on an important mission to reduce your weight and become healthier. Moreover, there will always be those who try to sabotage your diet whether on purpose or not. Don't let them. Your weight loss diet is too important.

Excuse 57 - I Live To Eat, Not Eat To Live!

I guess this is your philosophy to life. We should enjoy life. However, I suspect such thinking has gotten you overweight. In addition, the premise is not entirely true. You do eat to live or you wouldn't eat at all and you wouldn't live. Eating isn't life. Your life is more than eating.

There are major players in the diet world who in fact, have just the opposite philosophy. They believe you should eat what helps you live a healthy life. Dr. Joel Fuhrman's diet "Eat to Live" is one of the most popular diets. His diet is all about eating healthy foods that enhance your life and wellbeing.

I imagine this excuse comes from somebody who hasn't any plans to go on a weight loss diet. However, if you're overweight the theory is a product of your misguided philosophy of anything goes.

Though being overweight doesn't necessarily mean a shorter life, there are few fat old people.

Love to eat foods that are good for you and toss in a treat now and then.

Excuse 58 - Hamburger and Fries - Meat and Vegetables

Hamburger and fries, I mean meat and vegetables, and carbs, sodium, fat, and calories. MacDonald's new Grand Mac has 860 calories, 470 from fat, 1470 mg of sodium, and 52 grams of carbs. Add large fries, another 510 calories, totaling 1370 calories, which is almost a days' worth of calories, more if your allotment is 1200 calories per day. All that for one meal—not going to happen. Even if you're joking about the meat and vegetables, I see nothing funny if you are really trying to lose weight.

A homemade hamburger patty is 150 calories and a baked potato is 114 calories—264 calories total. There are plenty of jokes running around for dieters. I'm on a seafood diet. I eat everything I can see. If you eat something and no one saw you, it doesn't count as calories. Obesity is no joke. Scott Davis is a Christian comedian and often told jokes about his weight until he had to lose weight or else. Now he doesn't tell fat jokes. Being overweight is a serious health issue, which he and so many others deal with each day. Take your diet seriously and laugh off the diet jokes of others.

By the way, why do they call it hamburger? There is no ham in it.

Excuse 59 – I've Done Good

I've been good all week so I'm rewarding myself this weekend. I don't know how many times I did well on my diet all week and then just blew it on the weekend. I'd lose 3 pounds during the week and gain the weight all back and sometimes more on the weekend. Talk about frustrating. Losing a pound is hard but easy to gain one.

Now if you can reward yourself in a non-food way, great. Maybe a new book or a trip to the zoo. Some dieters make lists of things they want and set a weight loss goal to get them, a great way to reward yourself.

However, don't reward yourself with food. One large pizza can put you back a week. I know of no one who has rewarded themselves with a bowl of carrots. The reward is usually a food not on your plan you know you shouldn't eat because it triggers more eating off plan. One little cheat leads to another and down the slippery slope you slide. Don't use a cheat meal, or a cheat day. They just don't work in the end, one-step forward and two steps back. Just keep doing well on your diet, week in and week out. The best reward is losing excess pounds and becoming more active and healthier.

Excuse 60 - I Need a Treat

Yes, me too. Our body is always complaining because we don't feed it the Twinkie or an ice cream bar any more. Your body does not need a treat. Umm Magnum ice cream bars. There is no nutritional mandate your body will go into shock if you don't feed your mouth a brownie. The need for a treat is all in your mind. The mind is where the problem of weight loss resides. The mind is the battlefield for weight loss dieters, where you will fight the battle of the bulge.

The difference is between need and want. Your brain says I need a treat to help me overcome the terrible situations I faced today. Your diet should allow for a snack or a treat each day.

That said, there are healthy, low calories treats designed to help you through these "crises" situations. Fruit makes a good start. Our daughter makes healthy cookies. We have a pastor friend who has a little yogurt as an evening treat. If your diet is so restrictive you get no snacks or treats, then you may have a too restrictive diet. The body will crave things you are lacking in your diet.

However, your body is not craving a Twinkie because it is lacking what nutrition Twinkies provide—none. Most processed treats have no nutritional value. Protein makes a good treat along with fruit and nuts. Find healthy treats to calm your screaming body.

Let's face the fact, you don't "need" a treat, you just want one. I just went to the kitchen and the light was off. Charlene said the kitchen is closed. I didn't need a treat. I gave her this excuse but she said to go sit down and no treats for me. She made short work of this excuse.

Excuse 61 - I Eat Everything in Moderation

The idea is good especially if you are not overweight, but not a good idea if you are chubby. The theory is to eat whatever you want, but in moderation. Moderation is defines as "the avoidance of excess or extremes." Moderation is a subjective term meaning something different for each person. Therein lies the rub.

Some people think moderation is dieting during the week and eating what you want on weekends. Others say moderation is eating one piece of pizza instead of two or three or four. Generally, the weight challenged group see moderation as eating less of what you normally eat.

A diet can't survive on moderation. Eat what you feel is a moderate amount of chicken parmesan and put down your fork. Take 2 cups of green beans and put a moderate amount of light butter on them. Diets just don't work with those instructions.

The whole problem with moderation is we can't define the details. What I consider moderation you might not consider moderation. Moreover, let's face this head on, us weight challenged folk are not very good at going to the pizza place and eating one piece of a large pizza.

Everything in moderation is a common piece of healthy eating advice from slim and sexy celebs, dietitians and other lifestyle gurus. The idea of moderation is just not very helpful to overweight people, so just stick to your plan. If you are on the moderation diet and can lose weight then stick to the plan. However, I don't think it means one donut rather than two. As many experts agree, "moderation" may be ruining your health.

Excuse 62 - I Can't Find A Diet I Like

Most dieters are looking for a diet that allows them to eat anything they want, and sit and watch TV, and lose 10 pounds a week. If you've been looking for such a diet then you're right, you can't find one you like.

The whole subject of finding the right diet encompasses information beyond the scope of this excuse. There are plenty of resources available to find just the right diet to fit your needs.

I will be the first to admit choosing a diet that works for you is hard. I read the book and think this diet is perfect, and for whatever reason not so perfect for me. You need to do your research. There are websites giving reviews of various diets, such as Everydiet.org. I'm not sure how they base their reviews whether scientific, medical, opinion, or all of the above.

There are other websites as well. I've been a member of SparkPeople for years, and they have diet plans. There are websites that will plan your diet based on your input. If you have been dieting very long, you can probably come up with your own list of "diet foods" and create your own eating plan.

Decide what you want to accomplish with your diet. Do you just want weight loss? Do you want to combine weight loss with healthy eating? Do you want to add fitness in the mix? Many factors go into choosing a plan. Most people like a weight loss plan someone has prepared, with meal plans, food lists, and grocery lists. There are plenty of those available. There is a diet just for you.

Excuse 63 – It's Sugar Free

The Big Texan, in Amarillo, Texas, has a 72-ounce steak. If you can eat everything including all the trimmings in one hour, no charge. They cook a huge six-pound steak, all sugar-free. Sugar is a big problem in our society. Diabetes, which they use to call sugar diabetes, has to do with the regulation of sugar levels in the blood. Eating sugar-free is a good step forward in health and weight loss.

There are good sugar substitutes available, which replace the tons of sugar we eat each year. There are, however, concerns about many artificial sugar substitutes. I'm not going into those here except to say I believe artificial isn't good.

Another problem with sugar-free is we tend to think calorie-free when we say sugar-free. Russell Stover makes some delicious sugar-free candy. I was hooked on them when visiting my mother in California. She put them in her cookie jar. Still three pieces of the mint patties are 180 calories. Two pieces of Pecan Delights are 160 calories. Just because the label says sugar-free doesn't mean you can overeat them. Though going sugar-free is good, stick to your plan. Avoid any extra calories.

Excuse 64 – I Want a Diet Based On Science

The dictionary defines science as "the intellectual and practical activity encompassing the systematic study of the structure and behavior of the physical and natural world through observation and experiment." Is this what you're saying your diet should be? Do you mean a nuclear physicist should design your diet? I'm sure there is one.

What has science done for the diet world? Science has given us fertilizer, preservatives, colors, dyes, artificial sweeteners, artificial foods, confusing research, GMO's, and unpronounceable ingredients. For example, a single Twinkie contains 37 ingredients, but only five of them are 'recognizable', flour, egg, water, sugar, and salt. Twinkies' ingredients have fourteen of the top twenty chemicals made in the U.S. There are also five types of sugar in a Twinkie! Scientific research has been conflicting, and slanted to manufacturers.

Okay got that out of my system. Several diet writers say they use the latest science when designing their diet plans. Science is trying to determine the truth about various foods and diets. I use healthline.com/nutrition who say they have, "Daily articles about nutrition, weight loss, and health. They base all articles on scientific evidence, written and fact checked by experts. Our licensed nutritionists and dietitians strive to be objective and honest, and present both sides of the argument." They have a great deal of information on the latest research and make a conclusion based on the research. Good information and very helpful in deciding what diet to pursue.

Use the latest research to choose a diet plan. Just remember yesterday's science may not be today's science. Researchers are making advances every day and learning about the world of weight loss. Don't get too attached to a theory. Science would like you to eat a pill. Remember that overeating is the cause of weight gain regardless of what science may say.

Excuse 65 – Is It Recommended By the Government

I don't know if you are for or against the government by that statement. You may be thinking you don't want to have anything to do with the diet if the government is involved, or you really believe the government has good information regarding health and weight loss. Many see the government as health controversial group heavily influenced by lobbyists. You may be from another country and the departments may differ.

The US Department of Agriculture has a lot of information about nutrition and health. You might be most familiar with the food pyramid which displays government recommended food and portions. In 2011, they changed to the plate view called "Myplate" to simplify the Dietary guidelines. They have explanations for each of the categories. Many find this helpful although not especially about weight loss. They also have extensive food databases.

The US Food and Drug Administration handles the food labeling. I think they are trying to make the labels reader friendly and make sense. Various other agencies handle food safety. The CDC has helpful information on weight loss. The President's Council on Fitness, Sports, and Nutrition has many helpful insights into health and wellbeing. Nutrition.gov has a good deal of help in determining a diet and answer many questions on nutrition and diet. There is lots of free information in the government archives. Just search and ye shall find.

If you want a diet backed by the US government, you just have to read their dietary guidelines and adjust them to lose weight. They are just another tool in the weight challenged tool belt. Many experts out there in diet land don't agree with the government's dietary guidelines. So decide what you want from a diet and go from there.

Excuse 66 – I Hate to Attend Meetings

Some diets require you to attend meetings usually for a weigh in and a pep talk. Some require you to check in two or three times a week for weigh in and counsel. I've done them all. I remember one diet where we attended a meeting and if you lost weight, they applauded and if you gained weight, you had to wear a pig nose. Now there is meeting you could hate.

If you don't have time for meetings, then find a diet, which has no meetings. Some diets stress they have no meetings. However, I have observed meetings do help. They provide a measure of accountability. I have found them to be nonjudgmental and provide helpful tips when the diet isn't going so well. I have also found many reward weight loss in various ways, including recognition such as your name on the white board. Some will include recipes and food tips for putting variety in your diet and still stay on plan.

Another way meetings help is the old saying "birds of a feather flock together." You will meet people who are going through the same struggles as you are. You are not on the weight loss journey alone. You will find comfort knowing other people want to reach their weight loss goals just as you do.

Meetings do help, so go, don't hate.

Excuse 67 – I Don't Want To Be Accountable To Anyone

Dieters who are not accountable to anyone will probably fail. I know the feeling of having to tell someone your weight each week, or saying you strayed this week. It is embarrassing because you feel so weak. However, the opposite will happen if you do have to confide in someone each week.

You need someone or a group to make you accountable. This is a good thing. I found that when I had to weight in I worked harder to lose the weight so I wouldn't look so bad. I wanted to show I'd stuck to the plan and the plan worked for me. The first couple of times, you might get a little antsy over weighing in front of someone, but you get over it rather quickly.

Find someone you can be accountable to and make it a consistent check-in. If you really want to lose weight, make sure you aren't doing it alone. Find a group of likeminded people who are trying to lose weight and have a weekly check-in. Some diet plans have check-ins. Be accountable to someone in order to promote your weight loss success. If you really don't want anyone to know you are trying to lose weight, then chart your progress and be accountable to yourself. Keep the chart moving in the downward direction.

Excuse 68 - Regular Meals Are Impossible

In today's society, I'm not sure what you mean by regular meals. If you mean where the whole family sits down at the table all together, I agree normal is becoming more difficult. If you mean you are on the go and never seem to be able to stop and sit at a table and eat, then you might have to define "table" a little differently.

Most diets allow for three meals and three snacks, which means eating a breakfast, which could consist of a smoothie, for example. Most experts agree breakfast is important. You need to fuel your morning. Lunch may be at home, work, at a restaurant, from a bag, or maybe even on the road. Dinner may be the same depending on your schedule.

Weight loss dieting requires flexibility. I worked later shift hours many years, requiring a very different schedule for eating and sleeping. Flexible eating is the new normal eating. Although consistency helps in the weight loss diet, it's not always possible. However, eating on plan is always possible. I took my snacks and lunch to work in a cooler each day no matter what shift I worked. I walked during my lunch hour after eating. Maybe regular meals are no longer an option, but should never be an excuse not to eat according to plan.

Excuse 69 – There's Nothing in the House to Eat

Wow red flag. I don't know how many times I've had the same excuse. I've even dug into the raw oats cereal box with a spoon. I call it an act of rummaging. You don't want to be on a weight-loss diet and be rummaging. If you are hunting food, then there could be an emotional element to handle, or you might be a little hungry.

Now we are assuming you purchased your weekly groceries to fulfill your diet plan. If you haven't, what are you waiting for—go shopping. However, don't buy any food not on the list. If you do, you will find something when you go rummaging and in fulfillment of another excuse. In addition, don't shop when you're hungry.

When you go on a weight-loss diet, you will have to eat less than you're using to in order to lose weight. So you might feel a little hungry occasionally. Some diets want you to eat big salads so you are full. However, a salad doesn't last long, and you might go rummaging. Embrace the hunger. Don't eat any more than your diet allows. Be sure to eat all the food your diet allows. Nutrient dense foods also help, including protein. Make sure you get enough protein. I told my doctor I was going on a diet and she said be sure to get enough protein. Eat healthy. Don't go rummaging.

Excuse 70 - Healthy Food Is Tasteless

I'm not sure about this one. However, my guess is the person who said this was in the habit of eating processed foods. You've taught your taste buds to crave extreme flavors over the years—lots of sodium, sugar, and fat—gobs of processed foods, chips, cookies, crackers, and desserts. Then you start eating veggies and meals fixed with healthy foods and they seem bland in comparison. Squash, sweet potatoes and other veggies seem like eating tasteless foods.

Go back to eating real foods, and your taste buds will go back to their natural state where they will be able to discern and appreciate natural flavors.

You can also discover a whole world of spices. You can spice up the tasteless foods and make them zing. **When you stock your spice rack with a variety of herbs and blends, you're always ready to make a flavorful meal. There are perhaps thousands of spices in the world. Try some new ones.** Healthy food does not have to be tasteless.

There is an infinite supply of recipes on the internet. Go to a bookstore and there are shelves of cookbooks. Make it a conquest to prepare healthy and tasty food. You can easily overcome this excuse. There are plenty of alternates. Keep eating healthy and soon your tasteless food will taste great. Healthy food is tasty. So no excuses about food tastes.

Excuse 71 – I Can't Eat Beans or Some Veggies Because Of the Gas

This can be a problem especially if you are self-conscious. Everybody toots from time to time. The older you get the more likely you are to pass gas at an embarrassing time, but you are also less likely to be concerned about it. Gas is a natural result of the body's digestion processes. In general, gas occurs by how the body breaks down various foods. Some are not so easily broken down and may cause stomach distress and flatulence. Foods such as beans, lentils, asparagus, broccoli, Brussels sprouts, cabbage or sauerkraut, and other vegetables, dairy products, and some artificial sweeteners can cause gas.

If you are burping and passing gas often say 25 times a day, you may want to look at the foods you are eating. Yes, you may have to quit eating your favorite baked beans. Eliminate one food at a time to see what is causing the main problem. The diet I'm on doesn't allow beans anyway. There are also products you can take to relieve the gas. Don't let this be an excuse preventing you from losing the excess weight you're carrying around each day.

Excuse 72 – I'll Just Take One Bite

A chocolate frosted cake sits in front of you and you say I'll just take one bite. A plate of brownies is on the counter and you will take one bite. You go to an all you can eat place and say, I'll take one bite. I'm not sure why a skinny person would be reading this book because you aren't overweight. No weight challenged person can take one bite. Taking too many bites is why you are overweight.

Overweight people will recognize this in many ways. They order the biggest hamburger, the largest fries, the humongous drink, and fall for the get two more for just $1.

I had a friend who was working with a company who was writing manuals and one was on being overweight. The owner told him to review the draft, and he knew from dieting experience the manual wouldn't help because overweight people just don't stop eating when told to stop. The problem is much more complicated.

Why can't we stop at one bite? I've been here many times, and the answer is I don't know. Science tries to explain it with hormones. Psychologists, nutritionists, diet gurus, and other experts all have their theories, but to me they all fall short. Some say the problem is emotional, behavior learned in childhood, survival instinct, physiological, or a conspiracy brought on from alien beings among us. The reason might just as well be aliens. Nothing really tells me why I can't just take one bite.

This excuse is really just stating my weight challenged profile. I can't eat just one either. I can't explain it, and giving me quick fixes doesn't help much. It is a problem we have to face head on and try to minimize by avoiding the plate of brownies or the chocolate cake. I don't recommend facing your one bite problem by making a plate of brownies and just staring at them until you no longer have an urge to eat them. We became overweight by our lack of willpower.

We know this is a problem and very likely the reason we are overweight, so we have to handle the situation somehow if we are ever to lose weight. We can't however, let this be an excuse to overeat. We have to deal with the problem in some fashion and at the least minimize its effects. Since you know you can't just take one bite, you have to avoid these situations by not having any food in your house not on plan. Stay away from a plate of brownies.

Excuse 73 – It's Half the Calories So I Can Eat Twice as Much

I heard this one recently from an overweight person. Sounds good. The theory is if you can lower the calories, you can eat more. If you were at your goal weight, I would say go for it. However, the whole idea of losing weight is to lower the calories. The problem that got you overweight is portion control. Yes, you can't control your portions. Why eat twice as much and ruin the reason for buying lower calories foods.

It's a matter of renewing the wrong thinking and replacing it with new thinking. The old thinking was eat as much as possible and gain weight. The new thinking must be eat only what is on my plan and lose weight. Remember, to lose weight you have to cut the calories. So finding foods that replace higher calories is good. You got have the equation right—a food with half the calories. That should be your goal. It's half the calories so I lose more weight and still enjoy something I like.

Excuse 74 - I Blew My Diet

You mean you ate something not on your diet, or you just ate too much. From experience, you are going to stray from your diet for at least a lunch sometimes. My first thought is to just pick up and go from there. Splurging on lunch is not destroying your diet.

Maybe do some evaluating but don't be condemned or feel guilty about the indulgence. Assess your slip up and figure out what you could have done differently. Eat a lighter dinner and get back on track immediately.

My second thought is most diets today are so restrictive staying on them all the time is very difficult. This is especially true if you go out to eat or travel much. Most of us just want to get the weight off and then we can get back to normal.

Actually, any diet will get the weight off. Keeping it off is the problem. Getting back to normal for most dieters means going back to the ways of eating that made you fat in the first place. So pick an eating plan you can live with the rest of your life. If you fall off track for a lunch, move on. Don't go off track the rest of the week and don't' put off restarting your diet until next Monday, which would be a great hindrance to your weight loss journey.

Jack G. Elder

74

Chapter 3

Exercise Excuses

This section is about exercise excuses. Exercise builds health and endurance, and assists the weight loss process. Most good diets recommend some exercise from simply walking to full-blown gym workout routines. Although you can lose weight without exercise, the health benefits are worth the trouble. The idea of exercise does open the door for more excuses.

Excuse 75 - I Hate Workouts

Me, too. This implies you think you must go to a gym and go through a torturous workout to lose weight. Not my idea of fun. Weight loss is mostly diet. Even if you never exercise at all, if you have a good diet and stick to the plan, you would lose your weight. That said, am I saying exercise isn't important? No. Exercise has so many health benefits. This is especially true the older you get, and it doesn't have to be a strenucus "workout."

Exercise can be as simple as walking. Charlene and I walk every day we can, weather permitting. We have a treadmill and a recumbent bike for use when the weather isn't good or too cold, as today. We use walking videos inside when weather isn't suitable to outdoor activities. If you live near a mall, you can walk there when weather is too hot, cold, or inclement.

There is a myriad of ways to fit some exercise into your day's activities. When I worked, I would walk the stairs each lunchtime, which provided a good workout. Take a dumbbell to work and exercise while sitting at your desk. Maybe you don't like gyms or don't have the money for one. Look around. There are inexpensive gyms not requiring long-term memberships. Charlene and I participated in a yoga class. If nothing else walk, walk, walk. Turn your hate for exercise into at least a like and help your health and your weight loss.

Excuse 76 – Exercising Takes Too Long

In this age of instant everything there is no instant exercising. A one-hour workout is only 4% of your day, not much compared to the 96% you have left to do other things. The body takes time to get in shape and to stay fit. Your muscles take time to grow and heal and stretch and heal. There is no instant about exercise. In fact, learning the routines will take a little longer at the beginning, but you will soon be rolling through those reps.

However, there are ways to get a good workout in less time. Do a web search for 30 minutes even 15-minute workouts and you will see plenty of ways to get a good full body workout in a short amount of time. You might be interval training combining both cardio and strength training. There are even 5-minute workouts, which are intense but extremely efficient. You can follow these intense workouts with stepper, rower, spin bike, or treadmill for as long as desired. You can spend as long or as little time you want and still get a great workout. No excuses about getting fit takes too long. You have the same amount of time as anyone else so use a little for exercise.

Excuse 77 – I Don't Want the Pain

So you have heard the "no pain, no gain" theory of exercise. The saying dates back to the 1500s found in John Ray's proverb collection of 1670 as "Without pains, no gains." The idea behind the saying is you achieve nothing without effort, even suffering a little.

Exercise pain is muscle pain and normal, caused by overexertion. The medical term is myalgia. If you go to the gym and the trainer has you pushing the weights until you can't move, you are going to experience muscle pain. Microscopic damage to the muscle fibers will cause soreness. This kind of pain will go away in a few days and worked out in subsequent workouts. To avoid this type of pain, go slow at first. Don't be lifting the 50-pound weights. Do a shorter segment and rest. Fitness comes with consistent workouts.

Some kinds of pain can signal something is wrong. Joint pain, fractures, and other skeletal pain you should take seriously as an indication you should follow-up with a medical care practitioner. Don't push on, as this pain won't go away. Yes, you don't want this type of pain. Again, always consult with your doctor before starting any exercise program. If you have physical limitations, stay within those boundaries. Exercise can be fun if you use some wisdom and don't take unnecessary chances. That said from a senior.

Excuse 78 - Too Out Of Shape

By this excuse, you just told me why you needed to go on a diet. Get the weight off and get to exercising. If you are extremely overweight, you need to check with your doctor before starting any exercise program. He or she may suggest getting the diet going before attempting exercising. When you do start exercising, start easy. The CDC estimates 80% of people don't get the recommended exercise. The U.S. government recommends adults get at least 2.5 hours of moderate-intensity aerobic exercise each week or one hour and 15 minutes of vigorous-intensity activity, or a combination of both. Exercise or lack or exercise is affecting younger generations as well as adults. Stay active for as long as you can.

Another problem is defining what "in shape" means. The definition is different for everyone. I might be in good shape to walk four miles a day, but in no shape to run a marathon. Therefore, when you say you are out of shape, you have to qualify the statement. **If you huff and puff going up stairs, you are not in good shape, and might mean potential serious medical problems. The contestants on the TV show *Biggest Loser* were often very heavy and they were under the watchful eye of the medical staff but still did heavy exercising routines.**

There is the shape an athlete needs and a basic shape for the average person. In shape might mean a good body fat percentage, a good cardiovascular endurance level, and a weight at a normal level. Just think of the Dr. Seuss quote, *"You're in pretty good shape for the shape you are in."* Don't let your shape, whether pear, apple, or banana be an excuse for not getting the weight off. Some diets just recommend getting the weight off and light exercises are optional. You can get in shape along with the diet. Losing weight will really help. Again, an excuse is just that, an excuse.

Excuse 79 - I Can't Afford A Gym Membership

The average cost of a gym membership is about $40 to $50 per month, often after a membership fee and signing a two-year contract. Too much for me and since many memberships go unused after the first two months, a big waste for me. I've been there, lasting about two months and getting tired of going to the gym. Some gyms such as Planet Fitness charge $10 a month with no contract, more reasonable and affordable by most people's standards. If $10 a month is too much, then there are many ways to exercise without a monthly cost.

We walk on a city trail nearby our home every day we can. The only cost is the gasoline the car takes to drive there—less than 2 miles. We also have walking DVD's we can do at home and costs only the initial cost for the DVD. You can even walk around your neighborhood at no cost. However, only walk places, which provide a good measure of safety. Our neighborhood has no sidewalks so caution for cars.

You can also have a home gym. We have a recumbent bike and a treadmill. To be truthful we seldom use them. We have a complete set of weights and weight benches. Buy some weights starting with some light dumbbells and as you progress, buy heavier ones. Once you pay the initial cost, you have them for life. Some people, especially seniors, just use cans of vegetables or jugs of water for their weights.

Many exercises you can do don't involve equipment—squats, pushups, etc. You can find many on the internet. There are plenty of ways to get in some exercise without breaking the budget.

Excuse 80 – The Wi-Fi Is Down

A fitness trainer heard this excuse at a gym. The person walked out. Wow what an excuse not to exercise. Apparently, this person has access to a gym, paid membership, and now works out but because the Wi-Fi is down and she can't—what, listen to some music or check her emails. I don't use Wi-Fi at most places. I have a cell phone provider with unlimited data so just stay on regular cell phone reception. I will give her the benefit of the doubt okay she hates to work out without her Wi-Fi. Trudging on a treadmill can be boring and a little music, radio, or even TV does help.

This is a sad commentary on exercise because, she went to the trouble of going to the gym to better her health and fitness, and she didn't follow through. The benefit of doing the workout should outweigh the inconvenience of not having Wi-Fi. How many people do their workouts without the benefit of Wi-Fi? Do they complain? To me this is just one of those weak excuses to getting out of what you know you should do.

<u>Excuse 81 – I Don't Like To Walk</u>

I think God created us with two legs so we could walk. In the days of yore, people walked everywhere. Yes, they didn't go far, but they walked. There are many people for whatever reason can't walk. So walking is a privilege. My main source of exercise is walking. As Leslie Sansone says, "Walk, walk, walk."

Most of weight loss is diet, but using a few extra calories helps some. If you're between 120 and 140 pounds, 30 minutes of walking at 3mph burns 100 calories. If you weigh between 160 and 180 pounds, you'll burn about 127 calories in 30 minutes. Increase that by walking uphill or walking faster. You can almost double the calories burned.

So what don't you like about walking? Is it the long walk alone and never really getting anywhere? You just don't like the monotony. No place to walk? All these are but excuses. Walk with a friend or spouse. Use the time to plan, to think, to pray, to observe nature around you. Walk somewhere and back, such as walk to a coffee shop, have coffee, and walk back. I even play Pokémon on my walks.

There are plenty of health reasons to walk. It's cheap, and you don't have to have any special equipment. Be careful walking on busy streets, or when it's dark, but walking can open up a new adventure. Load a walking app and be competitive with yourself. Try to beat your record. Walking can be fun unless you're totally against fun.

<u>Excuse 82 - Exercise Makes Me Hungry</u>

Researchers in the UK have concluded exercise does indeed make you hungry, but the *overall* result will still give you a calorie deficit. The food-exercise equation is imbalanced. You may take an hour to burn 500 calories but only five minutes to eat them back. Should you skip exercise if a heavy workout makes you hungry and causes you to overeat? Maybe. Although exercise is very important to your overall health, weight loss is mostly about the food.

Three observations come to mind. First, if you overeat after a workout, then you need to evaluate the why. Is this just an excuse to overeat? Yes, you might be hungry, but you are usually hungry by lunchtime anyway. Just eat your regular portion. In addition, keep well hydrated during your workout. When you are finished, drink lots of water. Some expert trainers will suggest a protein smoothie to help the hunger.

Second, this is an excuse. By now if you have read any of these excuses, then you know an excuse is a bad idea. Don't make this an excuse to not diet.

Third, just eat fewer calories then you burned doing your exercise. Keep a calorie deficit. Exercise in itself, unless intense, is not going to burn many calories. So keep your eating business as usual.

Excuse 83 - Exercise Makes Me Tired

A good workout should make you feel like you can take on the world. A hard workout may make you want to rest a bit after. An extra hard work out or long hike may make you feel exhausted, but you should quickly recover. All this depends on what shape you're in. If you are just starting out, you might overdo your workout and deplete the body of all energy leaving you tired and maybe needing to take a short nap. Always start slowly. Don't overdo the first day at the gym or take a walk too long for your level of fitness.

Your body takes time to build up endurance and lung capacity. It's all about oxygen and getting it to the cells. If you run out of breath, you can't perform and you tire. If you are just starting to run for example, you don't start with a marathon. Start small. There are apps that help you train for events such as a marathon or a half marathon. Hey, there are apps for everything these days including walking apps. As a side note, in January 2011, the American Dialect Society named "app" the word of the year for 2010. We commonly use the word today and shortens the word application. Drink plenty of water and stay hydrated. Eat some protein snacks as needed. When we hike, we take protein bars to help fuel the walk.

If you are just generally tired, your diet may be wrong and you may be missing important energy producing nutrients. You may need a doctor checkup. Take a deep breath and say, "I can do this."

Excuse 84 – I Don't Feel Like It

Hey, this one I've used many times. Now there are two ways to look at this. First, you just don't want to exercise or walk today. Maybe you're in a bad mood or something has upset you. Okay. We all have days when we don't feel like doing anything much less exercise. However, the very thing we want to skip could be the thing that gets us out of the bad mood. Someone said, "You are one workout away from a good mood.

"When you exercise, your body releases chemicals called endorphins. These endorphins interact with the receptors in your brain that reduce your perception of pain. Endorphins also trigger a positive feeling in the body, similar to that of morphine." That endorphin rush is what will help your bad mood turn good, Take a hike and turn your day into a good day.

Second, you don't feel well. Maybe a cold or a touch of the flu and you don't feel like exercising. Well, don't. Get your rest. Take plenty of liquids and some chicken soup. You can get away with on your weight loss journey this one excuse. Try not to allow sickness to get you off plan. You can get over this obstacle and move on.

Excuse 85 – I'll Just Skip My Workout Today

Easy to do. It may be for legitimate reasons, maybe a schedule change or something, but instead of skipping how about rescheduling. You may not think missing one workout would make a difference. If you think missing one workout won't make a difference, you'll make less of a difference by not doing some exercise today.

What I have learned from my years of dieting and exercise is if you skip one workout, it makes it easier to skip two and then three. It's a slippery slope. Look at what Wikipedia says about slippery slope. "A slippery slope argument, in logic, **critical thinking**, political rhetoric, and **case law**, is a **consequentialist** logical device in which a party asserts that a relatively small first step leads to a **chain of related events** culminating in some significant (usually negative) effect."

Yep, one little seemingly inconsequential decision leads to a rather large problem. We call it the dieter's lament. You know the thing you wished you hadn't done because now it all seems to have come unraveled. I can hear your mind churning this over and saying, why is he making such a big deal out of skipping one workout. Because skipping anything in the weight loss journey leads to a skipping mentality. Skip walking today. Skip breakfast. Skip your weigh in. **Skip to my Lou, my darlin! Have a very good reason before you skip your workout, whether at the gym or on the trail.**

Excuse 86 – I May Be Fat but I'm Fit

I don't believe I've ever seen a fat marathon runner. The only fat athlete is probably limited to Sumo wrestlers who are also fit. However, for you my friend I really don't think such is true.

Excess fat increases the risk of suffering heart disease by 50% and obese people were also seven percent more likely to suffer a stroke. Overweight people are more likely to develop coronary heart disease by 28%. The list of health issues just increases for the overweight such as type 2 diabetes, gallbladder disease, osteoarthritis, cancer of the breast, colon, gallbladder, kidney, and liver.

This excuse is one that could cause you serious harm. You may work out some, or walk, which is a good start, but you can't be healthy with excess fat. If you would lose the weight, and maintain fitness workouts, I'll be the first to call you fit. Please don't let this excuse stop you from becoming healthy and fit.

Excuse 87 – I'll Find a Treadmill and Use It Everyday

Let's see, I have a treadmill in the basement gathering dust and a recumbent bike in the craft room patiently waiting for someone to hop on and ride. They have become a collector of stuff. In the beginning, I used them, but they quickly began to fall into disuse. Now I don't want to disparage the idea you want to get some equipment to exercise at home. My mother used her exercise bike into her 90's. I still intend to use mine. Honestly, for me, treadmill walking is too boring for me. I'd rather be out walking a trail.

There are many ways to make walking the treadmill less boring. If you're competitive, then set a walking record and then try to break your record. Watch TV. Listen to your favorite music. Listen to an audio book. Talk on the telephone to someone who is also walking his or her treadmill, maybe even a video chat. Put a walking through scenery video on and see yourself walking through France or Italy. Search on "making treadmill walking less boring" and you're find many ways to change up your walking workouts.

Before you spend the money on exercise equipment, decide if you will really use them. Are you one who follows through with their plans or do you drop out quickly? Check for used equipment. You'll find plenty. Some people will give it to you if you'll come pick it up. Don't make having a treadmill an excuse to lose the weight. If you buy a treadmill, use it.

Excuse 88 – I Just Need To Lose Belly Fat

Most of us men do. The belly is a good storage place for excess fat. So is there some exercises you can do to melt away the belly fat? Spot training doesn't work. You can do sit-ups until you collapse, but it's still not going to melt away belly fat. It may help tighten muscles but by itself not reduce belly fat. Maybe you are like the man who said they had 6-pack abs under their fat.

First, belly fat makes you at a greater risk for many health conditions, including diabetes, metabolic syndrome, heart disease, high blood pressure, and gallbladder problems. I had to have my gallbladder removed. I hadn't really thought my belly fat was a possible reason. My purpose here is not in finding your solutions for belly fat, but trying to eliminate your excuse for not dieting.

You belly fat will diminish as you lose weight. For more information on belly fat do a search on the internet. You'll have plenty of information to keep you busy reading for a long time.

Therefore, before you start taking over the counter pills with promises of melting away your belly fat, take a deep breath and save your money. There is no pill, no specific food, and no exercise specifically targeting belly fat. Get on the weight loss journey and see that belly respond to your good diet.

Excuse 89 – It's Raining

Rain falls on the dieter and the non-dieter. Rain just falls. Like the Wicked Witch of the West, will you melt in the rain? I hope you're not saying you can't go running or walking because of the rain. In the south here, we can walk most of the year although an afternoon thunderstorm is probable. Rain does present some problems, because often the rain mixes with electrical storms making walking outside unsafe. When the thunder roars, go indoors.

We are often in Florida in the winter, and there isn't much winter. However, in the north during the winter months, outside activities are more difficult. Yet there are winter activities in which you can get some exercise. Then again, you might say, hey, it's snowing.

The weather has no effect on eating unless you have a picnic rained out. The eating plan is 80-90% of weight loss. Cut back slightly if you can't exercise as you usually do. Plan alternates. If you are a member of a gym, you have access in any weather. Some people walk the malls every day. I usually put in my Leslie Sansone DVD and walk in-house when the weather is bad. There are plenty of ways around the weather problem. Therefore, when the rain comes down, say I'm going to do an alternate activity instead. Don't let excuses pile up. Excuses only affect your successes.

Excuse 90 – It's Too Hot

Here is another weather-related excuse. They are all the same with different solutions. I think most weather-related excuses have to do with exercise rather than eating. As we have said before, eating is the most important part of weight loss. You can diet, lose weight, and feel good if you don't exercise. However, fitness is part of the health paradigm.

Last summer when the weather was hot, we walked early in the morning two miles and by noon, we walked another two miles before the sun became too hot. There were days we skipped the noon walk because of the heat. I think a little wisdom goes a long way in deciding not to exercise when it is too hot. This is especially true for us seniors. There are alternates to exercising outside. If you live near a mall, they often open early for mall walkers. I knew one pastor who told his people who didn't have air-conditioning, to go to the mall and sit during the heat of the day. There are always ways around weather-related excuses. Search the internet for ideas. Join other groups at senior centers or swimming pools. The weather can be a problem, but has many solutions not excuses.

Excuse 91 – It's Too Cold

The previous excuse was too hot, and this one too cold. Sounds like Goldilocks. They are still weather-related excuses. I was in Chicago on a business trip when the wind chill was minus 55 degrees Fahrenheit. I have never been so cold. I had myself covered and fortunately didn't have to walk far, but the short walk was still extremely cold—freezing. Okay, for me too cold to venture outdoors.

I also have been on Scout outings in the snow. We placed our tents on the snow and did all activities outside. We were prepared and survived the weekend. Charlene doesn't do well in cold. We went on a hike in the Smokies when the temperature was about 17 degrees, and her body just about shut down. Cold is dangerous as well as heat, so best to avoid weather extremes.

Stay home and do your exercising at home. Walk to Leslie Sansone walking DVDs. If nothing else, just walk in place while watching TV. The point about weight loss dieting is to find a way. There is always an alternative. Don't make an excuse. Make provision for the problem. Obstacles will be common on weight loss diets. Overcome and succeed. No excuses avoids diet failures.

Excuse 92 – It's Too Dark

We wake up early and have to wait for dawn's early light to go walking. The trail sign reads "closed from dusk to dawn." We can't walk in the darkness. Years ago, we would get up early and walk in the dark in our neighborhood before work. I really don't recommend walking or running in the dark.

Is it too dark to eat? I don't think eating is a problem in the dark unless you haven't paid you electricity bill. In summer, there are more hours to exercise or walk. In winter, not so much. In fact, if you work, you might have no time to exercise unless you do so in the dark or you go to the gym.

A metaphor for walking in the dark is walking without understanding. You don't have light on the subject. There is plenty of information available about weight loss. Some, okay a lot, might seem confusing. However, you don't need to be in the dark about weight loss.

When thinking about weight loss, stay in the light, stick with the plan, and be fed up with excess weight.

Excuse 93 - I Walked Today

"I walked today." All by itself probably sounds good. If you walked then congratulations. We try to walk as much as we can. Walking is good for you. We have IHeartRadio tuned to our favorite Christian station when we walk. When the weather isn't good, then we walk indoors. So if you walked today, great. However, there is always a big BUT you can't us this excuse to eat foods not on your diet.

I might use this excuse from time to time, because we often park in the Starbucks parking lot and walk on the nearby trail. When finished walking we go to Starbucks. Hey, I just walked two miles, and my walking app said I used 280 calories. Okay, dividing a tall skinny mocha for 80 calories works okay. However, I can't have a piece of 400-calorie banana nut bread.

Whether we walk or whatever workout we do, we can't use any excuse to eat foods we shouldn't. Stick to the plan, and keep walking also. Both will assist the weight loss. When you get to goal then figure your exercise calories into your overall plan. Then you can have a treat. Meanwhile, walk, walk, walk.

Chapter 4

Mental Excuses

These excuses rattle around in your brain and fall out your mouth before you can say "oops." They are excuses of commitment and incorrect thinking about dieting and the weight loss journey. Some are myths and some just incorrect observations from the past or you just don't care if you're unhealthily fat. Once you have a diet plan, the mind becomes the battlefield where you will succeed or fail.

Excuse 94 - I Always Fail

This begins a challenge to some of our most famous weight loss excuses. "But I always fail." Of course you do. I can say you will on several levels. This is one of those excuses, which is a statement of your weight loss-dieting journey to date. You have always failed. You believe you will always fail because you have always failed at any attempt you have made. You are in the majority because 95% of people who diet will fail. I'm hoping you will change the percentage. If you're reading this, you haven't given up totally. Good for you.

"For assuredly, I [Jesus] say to you, whoever says to this mountain, 'Be removed and be cast into the sea,' and does not doubt in his heart, **but believes that those things he says will be done**, he will have whatever he says" (Mark 11:23 NKJV).

First, you have to believe you won't fail. What you say is extremely important. Words come from your "believer"—heart—and wrong believing leads to wrong thinking *and* speaking. Believe you can and put God's resources on your side to help you not fail.

Second, you have to eliminate the excuses you're making for failing. You keep saying you always fail so you set up a reason for your failure. You don't feel so bad when you fail again because you knew you would fail anyway. You don't have any expectations to succeed.

Third, get a plan and stick to it through thick and thinner. Make a lifestyle change to enhance your success chances. Develop a strong reason for losing weight and use the reason to get you through the mean times. This will be your last diet because you will not fail.

Excuse 95 – I've Been Told Dieting Doesn't Work

Do a search on the internet for diets don't work and you will get 25,600,000 hits (as of when I searched). This is weight-neutral, anti-diet, and Health at Every Size approach system of weight control. Actually, they take the emphasis off weight and seek to find a balance of health and size. The theory is if the standard diet approach doesn't work, (95% fail) then why are we blaming the individual and not the approach.

"With all of the research we have supporting the negative physiological and psychological effects of dieting and pursuit of weight loss; I find it unethical to approach nutrition counseling with the old diet/weight-loss paradigm" Natalie Katz, RDN.

I have to agree we have to modify or adjust the old approach to include issues causing obesity. Just getting someone to lose weight isn't enough if they will just gain it back. Been there, done that.

Other experts say diets don't work; we have to find a lifestyle of healthy eating which addresses health issues. They say don't focus on a diet but a lifestyle.

I do believe that overweight people have more issues than dieting itself can correct. We should examine those issues and develop solutions.

In this book, we are looking at excuses. We aren't looking at the approach to weight loss. I believe we need to get the weight off since most experts agree that excess weight is detrimental to your health. The fact that 95% of people fail at dieting, means we need to look at the different factors causing this failure. These factors are not simple problems but complicated and no individual is the same. Looking at the standard diet paradigm the weight obsessive view may not be the best approach for all people, whether a person uses the anti-diet approach, or a lifestyle diet approach, the concept is still to get the weight off. Taking no action is not going to solve the problem.

Excuse 96 – I've Tried Them All

For me this wasn't so much an excuse as a statement of fact, a badge given long-term dieters. I've been part of diet websites with group threads for decades and one of the statements I've often seen is this excuse. Sometimes it isn't really an excuse but the fact for whatever reason the diet didn't fit. I really don't think we've tried them all because there must be hundreds of them.

The cycle of dieting, losing some weight, regaining the weight, and feeling guilt and shame, then starting a new diet is the standard diet paradigm. Part of the problem is the diet industry's approach to keep you coming back for another diet. You get to be a professional dieter who is just trying out the latest diet.

The earliest diet I remember trying was the Scarsdale diet. Developed in the 1970's as a high protein diet, and tended to work better for me in losing weight. I don't remember much about the diet or the result, but Scarsdale paved the way for many diets to follow.

Not every diet fits everyone, so the reason why there are so many diets out there in diet land. There are many reasons why certain diets don't work, but eventually we can't stick to the diet. We begin to find excuses about the diet. Many are legitimate. The diet is too expensive, too complicated, too unhealthy, too boring, or too not me.

Mostly, diets eliminate fattening foods in order to lose weight. We like those fattening foods so we don't care for restrictions in our lives. Most diets will help you lose weight if you stick to them. However, not all diets fit your diet style. Weight loss is too important, a diet out there will work, and I'm sticking to the plan.

Possibly, you need a very different approach to weight loss. Maybe you need help from nutritionists who approach weight loss in an anti-diet manner. Before you start another diet, ask yourself what you need for successful weight loss. Maybe you need counseling to overcome some pressing issues keeping you from weight loss success. Look for an answer to your needs. It may not be the standard diet. Our daughter, a holistic health practitioner, approaches weight loss from a holistic standpoint. Diet is just part of getting your health back.

Excuse 97 – It's Too Hard to Diet

I agree. If dieting were easy, there would be no overweight people. Most people fail. However, "too" hard is saying impossible and dieting is not impossible. I'd call dieting hard because weight loss goes against all the reasons, which got us fat in the first place. Dieting goes against unlimited pizza, and Big Mac's and French fries.

In order to lose weight, you have to eat less than what your body wants. Your body has built-in mechanisms trying to keep functions stable and normal. Dieting challenges those mechanisms such as cravings, fake hunger, feeling weak, and slowing down the body's metabolic functions. Your mind goes berserk and then the battle wages.

Part of the problem is your thinker. How you think about dieting will greatly affect your diet process. When you are in a place of rest, you will find the burden of weight loss lifted and you move to living a lifestyle of weight loss, which becomes part of how you live each day. Think of dieting as a way to meet your weight and health goals, something you can do. I can say from experience, dieting is not always hard. You will experience some hard times yes, but get into a groove with your eating and stick to the plan. Weight loss becomes who you are and what you want to be.

Excuse 98 - I Just Can't Lose

Didn't your mother ever tell you there is no such word as "can't?" Can't means "to be unable or not allowed to." I know there are a few people who for whatever reason are not allowed to lose weight. I've heard of husbands forbidding their fat wives from losing weight. Even then, you can still diet on the sly. The situation is unfortunate but rare. I know, what you are really saying is you are unable to diet. There is the possibility of a medical condition, which might make you unable, at least temporary. However, the excuse is you tried but were unable to lose weight.

I'm sorry but I don't believe you. If you stick to most diets, you will lose weight. I suspect you didn't stay the course but instead ate the course. Hey, someone has to say it. Maybe a diary of your food will reveal whether you are sticking to the diet and whether you are still eating too much. Some people struggle with this and fail because they can't get a handle on the diet and overcome the weight loss obstacles.

In a snippet from a book *Diet and Health with Key to the Calories* by Lulu Hunt Peters, A.B., M.D. written in 1918 she has this is part of a dialogue with imaginary characters.

Mrs. Weyaton

"We have heard you say that fat people eat too much, and still we eat so little?"

Me Again

"Yes, you eat too much; *no matter how little it is*, even if it be only one bird-seed daily, *if you store it away as fat*. For, hearken; food, and food only (sometimes plus alcohol) maketh fat. Not water—not air—verily, nothing but food maketh fat. (And between you and me, Mrs. Weyaton, just confidential like—don't tell it—we know that the small appetite story is a myth.)"

Dr. Peters is one of the first to state calories are important in the weight loss effort. In addition, interesting enough this was a problem back in 1918. If the truth were told, you are not saying you can't, but you don't want to, and that's a completely different excuse. Now when you get down to your last few pounds, you may struggle some to lose the weight. Time and persistence will win the battle of the bulge.

Excuse 99 – I Can't Commit

Again, there is the word "can't." I can't stand to hear the word. However, we will focus on the word commit. I realize there are many people who have a hard time committing to anything—relationships, jobs, and diets. I can't cover the huge topic of commitment here. You may even require some counseling to understand why you can't commit. Some people just feel freedom through no commitments. Sometimes carefree is good, for example, no debts. However, when the subject comes to excess weight, the noncommittal attitude can leave you in a sour place.

There are many reasons why people might not want to commit to a restricted eating plan. I get that. Weight loss is a personal choice. Weight loss requires a great deal of personal commitment to see results. You can't just "give it a try" without fully committing to the process. You will just be another statistical failure. People with long-term weight challenges have to commit to a long-term solution. Reaching your weight loss goal doesn't mean your days of commitment to weight loss are over. The weight loss journey is a life commitment for most of us weight loss challenged people.

When you say you can't, you mean you don't want to commit. You have to decide if your noncommittal ways have caused you to lose out in life and to lose out in your weight problems. Lots to think about in making a commitment to weight loss.

<u>Excuse 100 - I Just Can't</u>

Okay, how many times will we hear the "I can't" excuse? I would rather hear you "can't" come up with a good reason to put off losing weight. I know there will be many people who just won't lose for many reasons and will just die fat. They would rather not have to go through the mental torment over a long-term weight problem.

If you are more than 100 pounds overweight, I urge you to take action. Even though I don't like the idea, you might fit the surgery format. I know several personally who took the surgery route and have done well. I know a couple of people who haven't done so well. Surgery can always have complications. However, I think getting the weight off is important for your quality of life. Have you watched any of the TV programs about the morbidly obese dealing with their weight, those weighing over 600 pounds? That limits the quality of life.

Weight loss is a choice. To me, however, losing weight has never been a choice. I needed to lose weight so I had to. Everyone is different and has different goals and purposes to their life. Maybe being fat is not a problem to you. In that case, don't even try. It's not you can't, it's you won't.

Excuse 101 - I Can't Make Up My Mind

Doing nothing is easy. Procrastination is doing nothing and that's what most people do. You are in control of your mind. At least I hope you are. You decide what to do and do it.

Start with a reason. Why should you lose weight? If you can't think of a good reason, then you should tell your mind no I'm not going to lose weight. Do a search on reasons to lose weight. You'll have an evening of reading. From a quick perusal, I would say there are two basic reasons, health, and appearance. Health we know about. I've already mentioned the health problems overweight can have.

There is also looks. Do you have a closet with one section for your fat clothes? Do you wish you could slip into those skinny jeans and flaunt your skinny self through the mall? Even though it is probably unethical, would your boss consider you for a better job if you were thinner. Do your grandkids run off and leave you alone in the park trying to catch up. There are as many reasons for losing weight, as there are people who need to lose weight. Make up your mind—now.

Excuse 102 – The Time Isn't Right

Solomon once said, "He that observeth the wind shall not sow; and he that regardeth the clouds shall not reap" (Ecclesiastes 11:4). If you are waiting for the perfect time then you will be waiting a long time.

Waiting for the perfect conditions means you will never get anything done. This applies to life in general as well as weight loss. Perfect conditions do not exist. If you're waiting for when you will have enough time, money, and friends, etc. it just never happens. Not all the external contributing factors will line up at the same time. If you are a mother with kids, and your excuse is I have to wait until the kids are in school, then you have to remain fat until they are all in school at least 5 years. Then what? You need a job. You have to wait until the kids get out of High School. Do you see the thinking here? What about you and your quality of life. The time to lose the weight is now. Don't put it off until some Monday in the future when you finally have everything in order.

Excuse 103 - I Have No Willpower

Me neither. At least for most of us weight loss people, willpower wanes rapidly especially in face of a brownie. The "will" according to the dictionary is "the power of control over one's own actions or emotions." This is the weak link for weight loss dieters. The will is the mind's decider. The will says "yes" or "no." Some people do have stronger dispositions than others do. Our daughter, for example, has a stronger will than I do. However, people who are weight challenged already have willpower issues so the likelihood of having a strong will is nil.

Jesus said, **"Watch ye and pray, lest ye enter into temptation. The spirit truly *is* ready, but the flesh *is* weak" (Mark 14:38).** The flesh is the physical—mental part of us. When food temptations come along, we just don't have the willpower to overcome on a long-term basis. For many dieters after three days, there is no willpower left to carry on. We have to reach deeper. As Christians, we have the full power of God within us to overcome. We need help to carry on a weight loss diet. Jesus says to pray and receive the strength to overcome the temptations, which come with dieting. Lean on the Spirit who empowers us to stick to our diet plan. Don't count on willpower.

You need a reason to lose weight stronger than willpower. When your resolve fades then pull in the reason and empower yourself to continue. Whether health or your desire to play with Grandkids, you have to make the reason stronger than your willpower. You can make it through the mean times.

Excuse 104 – I Can't Overcome the Temptations

Jesus said, "Watch ye and pray, lest ye enter into temptation. The spirit truly *is* ready, but the flesh *is* weak" (Mark 14:38). I'm not sure if Jesus had weight loss in mind, then again, He is concerned with what concerns you. I cannot leave food out on the counter, especially desserts. My family was here visiting recently and bought some pizzas and put them on the counter. I walked in opened the box and took a slice. I had already eaten dinner but pizza is a temptation for me. By the way, I took a second piece later.

Yes, food temptations are difficult to handle for weight challenged people. It's part of the reason we are overweight. Temptations are out there everywhere. Go to the grocery store and the snack foods are on the ends of the aisles so you can't miss them. The coffee shop has snacks all over the counter and in the display case in front of you. A restaurant may even have a display of desserts in a rotating carousel. There are plenty of food temptations everywhere.

The best way to avoid temptations is to avoid the places where displayed. Don't put anything on the counter. Don't go to coffee shops/bakeries. Flee from temptation. You have to minimize the temptations. They aren't going away. Just say, I don't need that cookie. I'm losing weight, and I don't need the slice of pizza. Talk to yourself and tell yourself what for. Don't let temptations ruin your diet success.

Excuse 105 – I've Been Overweight All My Life

Then now is really the time to do something about your weight. There are so many health issues for overweight people. Creaking joints and hearts giving out, just to mention a few. If you have been overweight all your life, you probably have already seen negative health issues because of excess weight.

Now if you're saying this excuse, meaning my life will always be this way for me, then you have to search deep and ask is being overweight the way you want to be. You can't let your past control your future. You can't let what you are today determine what you could be. You have put up with being overweight all your life. Maybe you have even tried to lose weight but just gained it back. Now you have just given up hope of ever getting the extra weight off. Nothing is impossible, as you believe.

It is possible to change your life whether weight or anything else. You first have to renew your thinking. You have been thinking, "That's just the way it is." Being fat may be the way for you today but doesn't have to be tomorrow. Nothing ever changes with the idea this has always been a certain way. Just ask church leaders. Change isn't always easy but not impossible, and with improved thinking, change can be enjoyable. What do they say, "there are three things that are certain in life: death, taxes, and change. You can't avoid change, it's mandatory, progress however is optional." You decide whether you want change or not. If you don't then your excuse will rob you of being able to live a completely new lifestyle.

Excuse 106 – I'm Big and Beautiful

Big and beautiful, those two words don't seem to go together. We have all seen the plus sized models taunting their excess pounds as beautiful. These models are no doubt pretty and I understand the concept of accepting everyone for who they are. However, we aren't what we look like. Our size and looks are not us. We are really the inner person and beauty does truly come from within. We can't let the media define who we should be.

I also understand young people need to see a variety of body shapes in media and advertising, rather than just perfectly sculpted models. The norms we often see are unrealistic and unaccepting to people with any limitations. We are not all models.

However, we can't sweep obesity under the rug or put it in plus sizes to diminish the growing problems being fat presents. I see the heavy models and know somewhere down the line they are going to suffer the consequences of the excess fat. However, not everyone has to be a size 2.

I believe in no condemnation no matter what size you are. Many say we shouldn't use the term "fat" because the term is not accepting and puts people into derogatory categories. They say we should accept fat as normal for many people. I do believe we should accept everyone for who they are. God loves everyone equally and so should we. However, fat acceptance should involve taking personal responsibility for our fatness, not in shaming others, because people can choose to be the weight they want, but taking responsibility does mean putting an end to all the excuses. Everyone is beautiful but obesity is still the important issue of health no matter what we call people and how we accept them.

Excuse 107 – I'm Large Framed

Before I say baloney, let's see how to determine frame size. Determine body frame size by a person's wrist circumference in relation to his height. Measure the wrist with a tape measure and use the following chart.

Women:
    Height under 5'2"
        Small = wrist size less than 5.5"
        Medium = wrist size 5.5" to 5.75"
        Large = wrist size over 5.75"
    Height 5'2" to 5' 5"
        Small = wrist size less than 6"
        Medium = wrist size 6" to 6.25"
        Large = wrist size over 6.25"
    Height over 5' 5"
        Small = wrist size less than 6.25"
        Medium = wrist size 6.25" to 6.5"
        Large = wrist size over 6.5"
    Men:
    Height over 5' 5"
        Small = wrist size 5.5" to 6.5"

Medium = wrist size 6.5" to 7.5"
Large = wrist size over 7.5"

Okay now you can use this excuse if you're large framed—not. If you're overweight, frame size makes no difference. Too often overweight men use this excuse to carry around far too much weight. If you are large framed your goal weight would rise a proportional amount. For example, the average 6 ft. man should weigh from 140 to 177 lbs. You can lean to the higher end if you are large framed. You are not a 300 lb. NFL lineman. (You wouldn't be reading this if you were.) Therefore, toss this excuse in the hoop because it won't fly.

Excuse 108 - It Takes Too Long

Remember a diet is what you eat. A weight loss diet is a diet you are doing until you get your weight off, and from there on, we call your diet a maintenance diet. Therefore, you must get your head around the fact you are on a diet for the rest of your life. If you are overweight, then you will have to be on guard the rest of your life. You will never be able to eat the same as you did before you went on a diet. Dieting doesn't take too long because guarding your weight is forever.

Nevertheless, I'm sure this excuse is about the weight loss phase, which most people consider the diet. Depending on the weight you need to lose, the weight loss phase could take quite a while. Men lose a little faster than women do. Heavy people lose faster at the beginning. Experts say two pounds a week would be safe. One pound is realistic. How long is "too long" for you? You need to lose 50 pounds in three weeks for a reunion—sorry not going to happen. There is no instant weight loss. I have seen people needing to lose over 100 pounds and the weight loss process takes more than two years. When they reach their goal, do you think they thought about how long the diet took? Lose the weight regardless how long reaching your goal takes. You will think losing the weight was worth the effort.

Excuse 109 - Dieting Isn't Fun

Dieting isn't a party if that's what you mean. Is everyday eating fun? Could be, depending on how you look at life. People who say dieting isn't fun will also say work isn't fun, going to church isn't fun, and going to the relative's house for Thanksgiving isn't fun. Most of life, to them, isn't fun.

The dictionary says fun is "amusing, entertaining, or enjoyable." Amusement fun is going to Disney World, or going to the beach for vacation. However, the last word—"enjoyable" can fit most areas of life if you see life as enjoyable.

You are only going to be here once, and for a relatively short period. If you take life in general as a "pain in the neck," then yes, you won't find it enjoyable. However, if you look at life as a gift and you are here for a purpose and to enjoy your time here, then you will find work, church, going visiting, and yes, dieting enjoyable. Celebrate each phase of your life. When you go on a diet, receive the plan with joy and thanksgiving as you would with any meal. It's all good. Enjoy the process, you will find yourself in a much happier place. The secret to losing weight is having fun while walking the journey. Find the fun in life and find the fun in weight loss. Watch that scale back down.

Excuse 110 - I Get Harassed For Dieting

This is one of the most unusual excuses because you'd think this excuse would never come up. However, it happens, I don't mean just Aunt Edna who wants to overfeed you and says you're so thin. Although family is often a source of hassle for the dieter, I've also seen this in the workplace. I can't understand the rationale because you'd think people would want you to lose weight and gain your health back, but is not always the case.

I think this aggravation comes from other overweight people who know they should be on a diet and you being on a diet just makes their problem even worse. They know they should be on a diet but for whatever reason aren't and now you are making the right move and are on a diet. Instead of going on a diet themselves, the easier path is to try to get you to go off your diet so they can say, "see diets are impossible." You are telling them you think dieting is possible and they resent your effort.

Sometimes I think you might be better off if you didn't announce you were on a diet. Just lose the weight. When they start asking if you lost weight or something, then you can proudly say, "Yes I have." Don't let others sabotage your weight loss efforts. Stick to your plan and you will have the last laugh.

Excuse 111 – It's Easier to Just Give an Excuse

Excuses undermine your whole way of life and this is particularly true for weight loss. Weight loss dieting is difficult. You have to give your whole being—body, soul, and spirit—working in full cooperation and unity to make the whole process a successful endeavor. Over 95% of people don't make it, which means to be one of the 5% who do make the goal you have to be strong. You don't need excuses, which are going to weaken your resolve to win at weight loss. Excuses just make you weak.

This isn't only true for weight loss but every area of your life. Every time you say, "I can't" you weaken your possibilities. Every excuse cuts your resources to endure the troubles and temptations coming with weight loss dieting. You just don't need them. If excuses make you weak, then not giving excuses makes you strong. Positive thinking about yourself and about the new you will strengthen and is always good. Knowing God's Word on the matter will make you even stronger. His grace is sufficient. You can do all things through Christ. No excuses please. You don't need them.

Excuse 112 - I Blame My Genes

You would be better off blaming your jeans. You have had no part in obtaining your genes. You are the product of your parents, grandparents, and great grandparents. Whether you are tall or short, big-boned, or thin, male or female, you can't change what is and the past. Blaming relatives won't help your situation.

Adam and Eve were the first to start the blame game, Adam blamed Eve, Eve blamed the serpent, the serpent, well, he had no one to blame. You can't blame your parents for your inability to stick to a diet. Yes, they may have had some responsibility in your being heavy, but there's where the blame game stops. No amount of blame can change one fact; *you* have to change your life for the better.

Even though experts say your genes affect up to 80% of your physical attributes, such as weight and height, etc. you still control what you do with your life. Scientist say they have isolated a fat gene, which makes dieting impossible. I don't like the word impossible; however, genes for a tiny group of people may make dieting very hard. Yet look at this thought. Genes have been around as long as human beings have, but the current obesity epidemic is brand-new. Genes don't cause obesity. Yes, you might be more susceptible but your genes aren't going to make you overeat and get fat. Don't blame your genes. Take responsibility for your life and do what you need to do. Don't get caught up in today's blame game where everyone is blaming someone else for his or her problems. Take control of your weight challenges and face them head on.

<u>Excuse 113 - I Don't Have Time</u>

This excuse has to be qualified. Time is one of the most precious commodities we have, and we need to handle each minute wisely. Everyone has the same amount of time—24 hours a day. We sleep for 8 hours of sleep, leaving 16 hours. If you work and travel to work there's another 9 hours leaving you with seven. Eating takes an hour a day, now six left. Yes, the time available dwindles rapidly. If you have kids, add some playtime, and maybe school work help time, etc., two hours leaving four left. Most people spend the rest of their time watching TV. Therefore, time is very limited.

Dieting doesn't take up any extra time. You have to eat so you can't be saying you have no time to eat. I suspect you are thinking you have to spend extra time in the gym you don't think you have. Thirty minutes of exercise a day, will really help whether you work out at home, walking, or at a gym. I think you can do something.

You might need some more planning and time management. You might have to set priorities and change your schedules. Maybe less TV. Make use of a calendar. Write to do notes. Get your whole family involved in good use of time. Other people manage, and so can you.

So although time is precious, so is your health. Lose the excuse, and lose the weight. You have to make time for your health.

Excuse 114 - I Don't Have Enough Time

In the previous excuse, you didn't think you had time to diet, but in this excuse, you tried but didn't have enough time. Huh? Are you saying you didn't have enough time to eat? Dieting is just eating. Just buy the right foods, prepare them, and eat. Eating takes no additional time than what you're using now.

Maybe what you are saying is you couldn't find time to exercise. You think dieting requires a great deal of exercise. You watched *Biggest Loser* and saw how much time they spent exercising. Well, that is a controlled environment and is not for the real world.

First, you don't have to exercise to diet. There's no "law" stating thou shalt exercise on your diet.

Losing weight is mostly about eating anyway.

Second, there are plenty of ways to get exercise in during your day. Search the web for 5-minute, 10-minute, or 15-minute workouts. Move as much as possible during the day. Walk at lunch if you work. Take the stairs. Walk in place at your workstation. Stand and do your work. Take long walks on the weekends. The only way you don't have time is because you don't want to exercise. You are no busier than all the people who do their exercise. Take some time for you and reap the benefits for your time spent.

We make time for those things we want to do. Want to lose weight and you'll make time for it.

Excuse 115 - I Can't Change

Another "can't" statement. There is no such than as can't. However, I digress. We are focusing more on the change aspect here. The "can't" is self-explanatory. Although I could ask the simple question, why can't you change? Even old dogs can learn new tricks. Even the oldest dieter has made changes. The "can't" is more probably an "I don't want to change." Okay fine, you don't have to do anything you don't want to do. That's the way life is. Life will change no matter what.

There will be change to a weight loss diet. If you continue as you have been, gaining weight every year, then life will be as it is. Isn't that the definition of insanity? If you want life to be the way you are, then no use trying to change. If you want to be fat and unhealthy because of your weight, then continue as you have been. However, if you are reading this, you still have a glimmer of hope you can lose the weight, which so easily besets you.

If you want to lose the weight and to get in shape, and I hope you do, then something has to change. First, your eating habits must change. How you have been eating up until today has put on the pounds. Your diet must change. You must alter your meals to accomplish weight loss and not weight gain.

Second, your exercise habits must change, or both exercise and diet. Change is synonymous with weight loss dieting. A change of diet means just that—change. Now you can change a little at a time, or change everything at once. However, to lose weight you have to change the "can't" to a "can." There is no weight loss without change.

Excuse 116 - Dieting Takes Too Much Discipline

"I'm just not disciplined enough, okay?" Okay. Are you talking about "the practice of training people to obey rules or a code of behavior, using punishment to correct disobedience?" Well, discipline also means "a branch of knowledge, typically one studied in higher education." You might say then discipline is a discipline.

What do you mean by "too much?" Do you mean dieting takes a lot of discipline and you don't have much or are you saying you don't like discipline? Maybe you are an undisciplined person. If such is the case, dieting is going to be very hard. There is a certain amount of code for behavior to stick to a diet plan. Think of those people in various fields of endeavor who reached their goals. They all had to exercise discipline in their efforts. Olympic athletes, sports celebrities, actors, and musicians, all reached their goals by sticking to their plans.

Okay, I'm thinking you mean you can't stick to a diet because you think dieting requires a great deal of discipline. Dieting does take discipline. Discipline means sticking to the plan. Ninety-five% of dieters can't stick to the plan. I will be the first to admit dieting can be difficult at times.

However, discipline is lessons learned. The word discipline comes from the word disciple or learner. Nobody is perfect. We all have weaknesses we are working on. Most of us hate rules, but to lose weight there will be of necessity some rules otherwise we would be doing the same things we are doing with the same success—none.

Therefore, you can learn the ropes of a weight loss diet. You can learn your code of dieting so the punishment of fat won't come upon you. You may not start with much discipline, but you can grow into it. **"For God hath not given us the spirit of fear; but of power, and of love, and of a sound mind" (2 Timothy 1:7). "Sound** mind" means discipline. God has given you discipline already, so use it.

Excuse 117 - Dieting Is Impossible

Impossible is a harsh word because with God all things are possible. If you do a search on the fact diets are impossible to keep, you will get plenty of hits. Since 95% of dieters fail, I suspect 95% of people would agree dieting is impossible. Some even say losing weight is scientifically impossible, because the body will just not allow it. Our bodies fight us by making us hungrier and holding onto calories more efficiently. I have to disagree, because if anyone has lost weight then it's possible. Many have succeeded in losing weight.

I will be the first to say dieting is difficult and seemed impossible for me for many years. The impossible thing might be keeping the weight off once you meet your weight loss goal. Most people can diet effectively by cutting calories but most people regain the weight. I've been there. The more you have dieted, the more yo-yoing you have done, the harder for your body to know what to do. Some diets are so restricting they are almost impossible. In addition, if you are dieting on willpower, diets are practically impossible.

If you **think** dieting is impossible, you're right. You can never override your beliefs. Your beliefs empower your abilities. If you are trying to lose weight too fast, you will give up. Choose a diet you can live with for life, and then the odds are with you. If you rely on God's grace, nothing is impossible. You need a completely new way of thinking and believing. If you don't think dieting is impossible, it isn't. There is hope through the power of grace.

Excuse 118 – Gaining Weight is Unavoidable as I Get Older

Some people do tend to gain weight, as they get older. The

problem is losing muscle and still eating the same amounts. Although I have found I'm not able to eat as much as I did when I was younger. We lose about 5 percent of our muscle mass every 10 years after the age of 35. This means if you're 70, that you have lost at least 20 percent of your muscle mass.

Two points come to mind. First, the muscles need protein to rebuild and maintain. Therefore, be sure and eat plenty of lean protein in your diet. I remember telling my doctor awhile back I was starting a new diet. Her only comment was to eat plenty of protein.

Second, is to add some strength training to your exercise routine. Use light dumbbells and work the various muscles to help build or at least maintain your muscle mass. Gaining weight is common as we get older, but isn't inevitable if we do something about the eating. If you need help with weight exercises and you are a senior, just search out weight training for seniors on the web. There is plenty of help. Also, stick to your eating plan and cut the calories a little.

Excuse 119 – I'm Addicted to Food

This is probably true. This is more of a cry for help, than an excuse. Obese or overweight people rely heavily on food for many reasons. They are often simply addicted to food. Probably the worst case of diet problems is true food addiction or as some call the foodaholic, the term used for people addicted to food like crazy. Foodaholic folks LOVE eating. These are the hardcore foodies. Now some folks just like to try different foods and eat responsibly—the foodie, but an overweight foodaholic faces serious problems.

First, they don't think they have a problem. Like the alcoholic, they won't accept any responsibility for their bad actions because they don't believe they are bad. Can we say "bad "anymore or do we use another word such as inappropriate. Maybe actions aren't bad but poor. I digress.

Second, this person usually has to hit bottom before they can see they have a problem. This person will need help. They may need counseling for their addiction. However, like breaking any addiction, there is always hope. I believe a person who truly understands who they are in Christ can overcome any addiction, even food. If you have a food addiction, where you can't seem to control your weight gain, then you have to go to the throne of grace to find help. Don't let food control you, but you control the food.

Excuse 120 - All My Friends Are Fat

Do you remember what your Mom always asked you? If everyone jumped off the cliff, would you jump also? Dieting is not about your friends, but about you. I know there's the saying birds of a feather flock together. I also know there might be something to want to be with like-minded friends.

If all your friends are fat, then you need to find a few other friends who aren't. Fat friends are not good examples for your pursuit of weight loss. Doesn't mean you can't associate with your friends but they could drag you down. You can find some Facebook friends or weight loss website friends. I've kept in touch with several over quite a few years. We all have the common goal of losing weight.

A dieter might feel like an outsider as the subject of dieting only comes up as a negative comment or two. Be the dieter who makes a difference. True friends will stand behind your weight loss efforts even if they don't lose weight themselves. Overweight people tend to sabotage the efforts of dieters. If they can't lose weight themselves, they try to thwart the efforts of those like yourself who are trying to lose weight.

As the joke goes, since losing weight isn't working, maybe making all my friends fat will. Talk to your friends about weight issues in a non-judgmental manner. Discuss the problems of obesity and health. If no one goes on the weight loss journey with you, okay.

Make your stand and lose the weight. Only you can lose your weight, friends, or no friends.

Excuse 121 - I Gotta Be Me

Sounds like the Sammy Davis Jr, song. "I've Gotta To Be Me."

What else can I be but what I am.

As Popeye said, "I yam what I yam, and that's all what I yam."

Okay. I know we all are who we are. We can't be someone else. You are the only you like you. However, does the fact you are fat make you who you are—the fat girl or the fat boy? You're letting your dimensions dictate your identity. You are much more than your weight, height, or looks, at least I hope you are.

Don't be who other people think you should be or how other people would describe you. They aren't you and you aren't they. In addition, you don't have to be overweight. That is not you.

I think who you think you are will have a huge effect on your weight loss efforts. Your weight can make a difference in how you see yourself. Obesity is a health problem. You don't need health problems. See the thin person within—the thin man or woman. Don't let being overweight decide who you are. Be the real you. See yourself as God sees you—loved, blessed, and perfect. Be that person, and then you can lose the weight without guilt or condemnation. Go ahead and be the real you.

Excuse 122 – Food Is My Only Pleasure

I grew up in a church where they seemed to forbid everything except eating. I couldn't go to shows, dances, play with playing cards, read comic books, and go to bowling alleys. However, we went to many potlucks where we gorged on all kinds of pots of homemade food. Still then, I didn't think eating was the only thing left to enjoy as I still enjoyed my childhood.

Okay, I still enjoyed my years in school and I certainly didn't think food was my only pleasure. A person who says food is their only pleasure lives a very limited and boring life. Sunsets, sunrises, rain on the window, drive to the beach or the mountains, and so much more give me pleasure. Meeting up with the kids, grandkids, and great grandkids makes my day.

Sometimes a meetup involves food, sitting around a table or at a restaurant. The last time we visited the great grandkids in Texas, I spent a great deal of time playing with them in their rooms. I enjoyed every minute. That's why they we call them "great."

Broaden your outlook on life. Read a good book. Take a walk. Hike the nearest nature trail. Go to a zoo or an aquarium. Have a cup of coffee at a new coffee shop. Play games with friends. We have a large group of people who play Pokémon Go together. When you do eat, enjoy the meal. Life is a pleasure, so live it.

Excuse 123 - The Family Won't Diet With Me

Anytime I use the word diet I always mean weight loss diet. So we have to ask, are you the only one in your family who needs to lose weight? If so, then you have to diet on your own. Yes, you might have to fix two separate meals. However, you have to do what you need to do to lose the weight that is besetting you.

You can make most diets easily into family meals, such as meat and veggies. If there are other family members, who need to lose weight, then put them on the diet. Husbands can sometimes be obstinate. Fat husbands can be troublesome I know. Talk about the issues in a non-judgmental way and share the benefits of losing weight.

Suggest they can help you as well as themselves be healthier. If your husband is Archie Bunker, then fix meals they like and sneak in a few delicious diet recipes. Don't neglect yourself. Don't let this become an excuse for not losing weight. Weight loss is for you, and your family. You will have more energy and spunk to make it through each day.

Excuse 124 – I'm Too Busy

This kind of goes with our excuse "I don't have enough time." My first thought is, maybe you are **too** busy. Everyone has the same amount of time each day. Everyone fills his or her days with something. I know if you have kids, they can take up a great deal of time. If you have kids and work, your time will be limited. Again, we aren't talking about being too busy to eat. You have to eat. A weight loss diet is about what you eat. You need no additional time to eat right than to eat wrong.

Driving through a fast food place is convenient, but still takes time. Learn to make easy-to-fix meals. Carry snacks with you. Use a planner and pencil in your workouts. Find quick ways to make breakfast meals fitting your diet plan. Make big batches on the weekends. Use the crock-pot. Get your family to help. You might be crazy busy, but so are many others who still manage their weight loss journey. Dr. Oz, for example, must have an extremely busy schedule, but he still eats right and gets in some exercise.

Maybe you should write down everything you do for a few days and see if you are just wasting time. Look at prioritizing your time and making sure you get some time for yourself. You usually make time for matters, which are most important. Your health and weight are important. Don't excuse your weight loss to being too busy.

Excuse 125 – Dieting Makes Me Too Weight Obsessed

I've been there. Making up diet plans, counting calories, making sure I eat right each meal, making up shopping lists, reading diet books, reading diet articles, and searching the web for recipes. This is both time consuming and obsessive as well. Sometimes when your whole focus is on the weight loss, it does become an obsession.

I like challenges, and losing weight is a big challenge. However, I no longer do all the calorie counting and associated stuff, and just stick to a basic plan. I vary the plan when we go on trips and then get back on track.

For the truly weight challenged person, losing the weight is only the beginning. Weight will always be a trial. Keeping the weight off is just as big a part of the weight loss journey as losing the weight is. You need a completely new mindset about eating and living without the weight. We have to eat, so we don't need to be obsessed over losing weight, when we can enjoy a new lifestyle of eating to last a lifetime. Don't make losing the weight the focus. Make enjoying life with a diet plan that will keep you fit and happy for life.

Excuse 126 - I Don't Want To Buy New Clothes

This must be a man's excuse. I don't know many women who don't like to shop for new clothes. Weight loss is a good excuse to buy new clothes. Unless you were once smaller but gained weight and grew out of your clothes—you had to buy bigger clothes—and you didn't keep all your old clothes, you will have to get yourself a new wardrobe. You will have to get rid of the Moo Moo or rather Muu Muu as well as all those other frumpy looking clothes. Instead of clothes designed to hide your fat, you can get clothes to accentuate your new look.

I might give you the excuse "I can't afford new clothes." However, there are ways to get good deals on clothes. Unless you are a fashionista, you can find many good clothes at thrift places. Some places are higher end than others are. Many stores such as Walmart and Old Navy have good prices on clothes, and occasionally you'll find great sale prices.

To me losing weight should be a reason to say, I get to buy new clothes. Besides those old clothes are out of style anyway. Instead of the women's size 20, or men's size 44 jeans, you might have to get a size 10 or 36, respectively or even smaller—yeah. If the budget is your problem, buy a little at a time. Save your money and buy a new outfit. Your self-esteem will soar. You will be looking mighty fine.

Excuse 127 - I Just Had A Baby

Well, this excuse eliminates half the population. Alternatively, we could add, I'm going to have a baby. Most women gain a great deal of weight during the 9 months of carrying a child. Moreover, from what I've read, many don't get the weight off when the next child comes along, and you add on even more weight. Therefore, from a weight standpoint, the fact you just had a baby is a good time to get on a weight loss plan. Postponing taking action now is just asking for trouble. I realize there are some precautions. We've all seen the restraints for nursing mothers. So take precautions if needed but get the weight off as soon as possible.

The baby will consume much of your time and energy and exercising is low on your priorities. Though breastfeeding burns 600 to 800 calories a day, chances are you will eat more sitting around. Decades ago, doctors liked to keep women physically restricted after delivery—no more. Most experts say get to moving early. You should try to get your weight back off within 6 to 12 months. In addition, if you weren't at your designed weight before the baby, then get the weight off. Don't end up with three children and an extra 100 hundred pounds and blaming your weight on your kids or your husband.

Anything is possible. I'm amazed at some of the celebrities who have a baby and seem to lose the weight overnight. Of course, if you watch your weight during the pregnancy then you won't have so much to lose. Again, you can do whatever you need to do to lose your weight.

Excuse 128 - My Friends Made Me Do It

Oh yes, the Adam and Eve syndrome. Blame someone else, the easy and cowardly way out of any situation. You aren't in control of your hands and they just fling food into your mouth. Such as a "Little Debbie Devil Squares" just falls off the shelf into your shopping cart. Moreover, you are blaming your friends. You must not like your friends. Fess up. You just slipped up.

About what are we talking? (Who made up the rule that says we can't end a sentence with a preposition?) Back to the excuse. Who knows what "it" is, but the problem was probably a snack not fitting the weight loss plan.

Come on and take responsibility for your life. Better yet, take control of your life. You are where you are because you made it so. You will be where you want to be because you took action. No one is going to keep you from eating what is not on your plan. Maybe there's a potential job—hand slapping. He or she is a person who goes around with you everywhere and slaps your hand if you try to sneak a forbidden treat. They could also encourage you when you win the struggle. Hey, don't blame, so you can claim the victory.

Excuse 129 - It Benefits A Good Cause

I'm sure you've seen the Girl Scouts selling their cookies each year, their major fundraising campaign. The $700 million raised goes a long way to fund the Girl Scout programs. Some fundraising programs use Krispy Kreme to raise money but I haven't seen any lately. Years ago as a Scoutmaster, we would sell chocolate bunnies around Easter to raise money for the program. On our walk the other day, some scouts were selling potato chips. These are all worthy causes. However, for the weight loss dieter, they are a distraction. You are your greatest cause.

Getting the weight off and keeping the weight off is priority one. If you have to skip the Thin Mints this year, then skip them. If you want to help the organization, just donate the money and don't take the cookies. I know, easier said than done. I know because our son brought some home this year and I snuck a few (I love those Thin Mints).

There are many good causes out there, but don't let them steal from you, your greatest cause. These causes can come multiple times a year, so be cautious. Overweight people have a hard time eating just one cookie. You might say I only a bought a box, but one box mentality is challenging you and soon your weight loss program is not a loss but a weight gain program.

Excuse 130 – I've Got Kids

Are you saying you can't participate in a weight loss diet because you have kids? As an interesting side note according to the Census Bureau, fewer woman are having children, for many reasons. However, you have kids and you say they are your weight loss problem.

I will be the first to admit having children, especially younger children does take more time out of the day you can no longer spend on yourself. Exercising becomes a little more challenging. However, I see women on the local walking trail with their kids in tow. Some run pushing their stroller. Some just herd their children along. Everyone is getting exercise. Are you up to a challenge?

I know exercising with the kids is not easy to do especially if you have complainers. I see that on the trail also. The kid in the back with his arms folded and the mom shouting "come on." With good planning, you can get in your needed exercise. Teaching the children early exercise is important and will have lasting effects on them. Now eating presents another problem. If the children are already used to junk food, you will have more difficultly to get your kids to eat healthy. My daughter changed the eating with her whole family however, so I know anything is possible. You have to replace the junk food with good tasting healthy food along with snacks they like. Teach the kids to eat healthy. They won't have a weight problem later on. Don't blame your kids.

Excuse 131 - My Husband Will Leave Me

You're actually saying your husband said he'd leave you if you lost weight. Sayonara, adios, goodbye. Okay, my first thought. I know life shouldn't be that way, but I've heard of men who want to keep their women fat. I can't begin to understand such selfish thinking. Obesity is a link to all kinds of serious health problems. Why would your husband want you to have serious health issues? Jimmy Soul sang a song called "If You Wanna Be Happy." The song says to be happy marry an ugly wife.

Funny, but sick. Therefore, my guess is the husband wants to keep you fat to keep other men from looking at you. Either way, it a horrible burden to carry. Work it out. Explain the benefits of having a healthy wife, and take your husband along on the weight loss adventure. You need to lookout for your health.

Excuse 132 - I Attend A Lot of Parties

I'm guessing you are a single person without kids. You love the party circuit and enjoy mingling with people. I'm not sure what "a lot" might mean, but if you work, you mean weekends. If you're overweight, then watching what you eat might present some challenges, but you can overcome.

There will be a day coming when the party habit will get old, and you still have the weight you wish you had lost. I think you can still participate in party time, and lose your weight. Plan ahead.

Fit in the calories your diet plan gives you each day. Pick a plan, which enables you to be flexible. If you know ahead of time that you will eat party food, then eat light for lunch. Take some healthy snacks to the party to share. You will at least have good snack to eat and not go overboard. If your partying is at bars and restaurants, then you have a problem. It's an environment not in your control unless you take special precautions to eat and drink low calorie. Might be you have to slow down on the partying and get the weight lost.

For every excuse, there are plenty of alternate solutions. Make your weight loss journey a high priority and get people on your side to support you. You can lose weight and still enjoy your lifestyle.

Excuse 133 – I'll Think about It

No, you won't. Thinking is not doing. In fact, there is a long gap between thinking and doing. Now going on a weight loss diet is a big decision, requiring major changes in your life. You do have to think out a few things such as what is the correct plan for you and have a good reason cemented into your consciousness for why you should go on a weight loss journey.

Most people fail at weight loss, meaning you will probably fail also. Particularly if you have tried dieting many times before. Yes, I would put some thought into the decision. Thinking carefully about dieting is the first step in making your weight loss goals a reality and not finding yourself in the fail column.

Think about how losing the weight will affect your health. Think about how tired you are every day and how little motivation you have to get off the couch and do something fun. Yes, there is plenty to think about, but don't delay with a false "I'll think about it" which is really procrastination. We're talking your health, your life. Only you can do anything about change. Don't just think—do.

Just picture Rodin's The Thinker posing in his thinking position as a skeleton. All he did was think and no action.

Excuse 134 - I Hate to Lose

I would lose weight but I hate losing. Very funny. Do you mean you love gaining? This is one of comedic terms where losing is winning. Tennis great Jimmy Connors famously said, "I hate to lose more than I love to win." I don't like the term "losing." Maybe it's the word "lose" you don't like. Come up with another one. Fat removal, gain skinny, thin down, weight removal, skinny down, body redesign, slenderize, and I'm sure you can come up with others. The idea is losing is not always bad. So when you go on your weight removal journey, always think of dieting as overcoming. This is triumph over weight. Weight is bad, and losing it is good. Frances Hunter wrote a book called, *God's Answer to Fat – Loose it*. Let it go. Don't hold on to extra weight.

When someone asks you how much weight have you lost say, "I didn't lose any, I got rid of it." Too many people lose weight only to find it again. The weight is lost and gone forever.

I suppose there is some psychology behind using certain words over others. A rose by any other name would still smell as sweet. Richard Simmons refused to use the word "diet" because it contained the word die. He called it a "live it." In fact, he has a book called "Never Say Diet." Losing weight is sweet victory. Don't get sidetracked by minor matters. If the word "losing" bothers you, call any loss winning. Go on a weight-winning journey.

Excuse 135 – Dieting Is another Way Men Control Women

I'm not sure from whence this excuse came. About 30% of women are on a diet and 25% of men almost as many men are dieting as women. Therefore, I don't see how men are controlling women. More men might lead the food industry than woman might, but they want everyone to be on a diet. I know many women model themselves on photographic models who are young, attractive, and thin thus implying this is what men want. So men want women to diet to meet some exaggerated view of sexy women.

Possibly, you are a diehard feminist who believe men are the problem to everything. I just read where they asked a 106-year-old woman her secret to long life. She said to stay away from men.

Men might think women are the problem. Regardless, this thinking doesn't get the weight off. If your staunch beliefs are stronger than your desire to get extra pounds off, then you will remain overweight and fall to yet another useless excuse.

Excuse 136 - I Hate to Weigh - Scale

This is one of my favorite subjects. If stepping on the scale will keep you from a weight loss diet, then don't step on the scale. The important issue is to get extra weight off. If you stick to the plan, then you will lose the weight.

However and there's a big however, you really need to check your weight loss progress. You are on a weight loss diet. You need to check whether you are losing weight. You may be on a diet not suited to you. You may be cheating a little. You need to weigh in occasionally to get the whole story. I weigh every day first thing in the morning. Well, maybe second thing. However, if stepping on the scale is a traumatic event, don't step on the scale but once a week or every other week. If the scale totally freaks you then put the electronic gadget in the closet.

Regardless of the "I hate the scale" movement, the scale is just a tool to help you along on your weight loss journey. I think weighing is the best method and most accurate way to check your progress. The inanimate digital gadget is not going to bite you, not judge you, not condemn you, nor will it even congratulate you. It just displays how much you weigh now. Go ahead and use the scale. Just don't over use it. No more than once a day, at the same time each day and best in the morning.

There are other ways to test your weight loss, such as clothing feeling loose, measuring tapes, wellbeing checks, and other methods of determining you are losing the weight. The most important part is losing the weight. I'm starting the "I like the scale" movement. Step on the scale and join the weight loss revolution.

Excuse 137 – I'm Too Old

I guess you are really old then. For the senior, getting weight under control as soon as possible is an important issue. This excuse is about age. What is the best age to lose weight? When you get fat. I've seen a lot of old people but few old fat people. I have dieted for many years and I have found at an earlier age, losing weight was easier. Now weight loss is harder, for many reasons. I also know as you age you don't eat as much. I also know research shows the BMI chart creeps up for seniors. Being a little rounder is okay.

I'm in my 70's and I am still on my weight loss journey. I am still active and walk as often as I can. I think eating a healthy diet in the correct portions is a diet anyone can live on and should live on no matter the age. I don't do some of the things I did in my younger days such as play tennis. However, many seniors do. There are many seniors doing amazing exercise feats. The idea is to keep moving as long as you can. If you are overweight regardless of age, adjust your diet to get back to your ideal weight. Don't use age as an excuse.

Excuse 138 - What If It Doesn't Work?

Most diets will work if you follow them exactly. Some weight loss diets are easier to follow than others are. Some require special supplements or special foods. I've been on more diets than I can remember and some of them didn't work for me for various reasons. High carb diets didn't work for me. I found the low carb or higher protein diets work better for me. If you know this about yourself, then you can choose a diet, which fits your weight loss type. There are all types of diets based on your blood type, your body shape, personality type, and now DNA. You might fit into one of these diets and have success. If you don't know these factors about yourself, you may need to do some experimentation.

Low carb diets work for the majority of people. Even a weight loss diet that fits you won't work if you cheat. Diets only work if you stick to the plan. You have to tailor the diet to your lifestyle. If you travel a lot, then you have to consider the travel problem in choosing a diet. If your time is extremely limited, then chose a diet that has easy preparation and not long complicated recipes. My question would be to find out why your diet doesn't work, and honestly answer. You might need a different one. No shame there. You are your problem if you quit.

Excuse 139 -I've reached My Goal

If you have reached your weight loss goal, congratulations. Not many dieters reach their goal. Truly an important accomplishment. However, reaching the goal is only half the process. Many attain but few maintain. Therein lies the rub.

Dieters don't maintain generally, because they think the weight loss diet is over and can now eat what they want. They fall into old poor habits of eating and soon the weight is back on. Somebody should have told you from the beginning, dieting to lose weight is a lifelong commitment. This is especially true for us weight loss challenged where seeing a cookie causes you to grab it. Once you reached your goal, the challenge begins. Maintaining your goal weight is your next step in living without the excess weight.

This may be harder than taking the weight off. You can't drop your guard for a minute. Not many can say I lost the weight and kept if off for five years or ten years. Start your diet as a weight loss diet and slightly modify the plan into a maintenance diet. You get to eat more and maybe a treat of two, but you have to stick to the maintenance plan. Congratulations for losing the weight, now please keep it off. Don't be yo-yoing your weight. No roller coaster weight. Keep your weight consistent and steady. Weigh each day and if the scale goes up, then back to weight loss. Watch what you eat and avoid old habits, which made you fat. Don't be a gainer.

Excuse 140 - I Just Don't Care

You don't care about health, length of days, quality of life, friends and family, fitness, and finances. Many people just don't want to diet even if they need to diet. If the "I don't care attitude" is just for dieting, then fine; but if this is your general attitude to life then you have serious problems. You need help.

Life is wild. You are to enjoy life. If you have obsessed over your weight since you were young, I get it. You are just tired of trying to diet, keeping a mental calorie counter going in your mind, and feeling elated one day and depressed the next. No wonder you don't care about weight loss.

Like me, you have probably been on a hundred diets, learning new weight loss protocols, failing, and trying the next one to come along. Most diets are too restrictive. You can't eat any of your favorite foods. You are tired of carrots and celery. Sometimes I get to a point I almost hate salad. My suggestion is care about your life. Find a plan you enjoy. Eat a little less and exercise a little more. Fill you days with joy and love yourself. Maybe get a little weight off in the meantime.

Excuse 141 - Fat People Seem Happier

I'm concerned when people look at other people and think they are happy because they are fat. This tells me you consider yourself happy because you're overweight. If you're comparing yourself to fat people such as jolly old Saint Nicholas, I think you are making a serious mistake. The operative word here is "seem." Don't fool yourself into thinking this lie.

First, let me say happiness is not contingent on fatness or skinniness. You can be happy no matter your dimensions or your circumstances. In fact, replace happiness, which is happenstance on circumstances, with joy. The joy of the Lord is your strength especially during trying times such as a diet.

Each year there is a higher percentage of people who are depressed and unhappy. Many of them start using drugs, both legal and illegal. My suggestion is rather than using drugs to struggle through, allow the joy of Jesus to permeate your soul. Things aren't always going to go well in life. That's where you can rise above the circumstances and live in joy.

Second, ask yourself if you are happier being fat. You can't run up the stairs. You huff and puff just going to the mailbox. You feel condemned for overeating, and the prospects for your future are bleak. Some fat people will joke about life on the outside, but are dreary on the inside. Does this sound like happy to you? Rise above to happiness and look forward to a life less fat.

Excuse 142 - Life Is Too Short To Waste on Dieting

Sadly, life could be much shorter if you don't lose weight. Regardless, you have a certain number of years here on earth. In light of eternity, time here really is short. Okay then, sounds like you don't have a very good perspective on what dieting is. Yes, dieting is restriction, because you have to eat less than your body needs to burn fat calories. However, the weight loss journey can be a challenging adventure. I've always liked challenges. That's why Grandpa Jack plays Pokémon. I look at weight loss dieting as a challenge to overcome. Everyone wants to be a winner. Nobody likes to be a loser, except of course, in losing weight. If you go out every night partying, then I really can't help you. You have to decide what is most important for you.

As a senior, I wish I'd solved the weight problem early in my life. Weight loss dieting is not for everyone. Some people don't care about their weight, and eating and drinking what they want is more important. However, seems to me people who think that way have other issues to resolve. Moreover, weight loss dieting is no guarantee of a longer life. Being overweight will eventually cause health problems you might not really want to deal with later. No matter how long you live, live life at your God designed weight. Quality of life is important also.

Excuse 143 – I'll Never Lose These Last Ten Pounds

I read a number of message boards, and this is one of the most difficult parts of the diet dilemma. You will go through plateaus in your diet and you will work through them. Sometimes you will go a few days before the scales moves and sometimes a few weeks. Your body is adjusting to the weight loss. You might be frustrated but you work your way through the plateau and never give up because the goal is in view. However, for some reason, those last 10 pounds won't budge.

If you Google this problem you will find all kinds of reasons and fixes for the problem of those last annoying pounds. You might think your scale is stuck, but your body is doing everything possible to hold onto those last pounds. Experts call it survival. You need to look at your plan. Have you been sneaking in a few extra calories? You may have to reduce the intake a little. On the other hand, what about your exercise? Did you start good but are waning a little—maybe not walking as often or as much? You might have set your goal too low. Wouldn't that be nice?

Do whatever you need to lose those last pounds. You can do it no matter how stubborn the last few pounds are just keep going. See yourself at your goal and speak to those last stubborn pounds to depart.

Excuse 144 - I Can't Do It Alone

You may think you are on this weight loss journey all alone. No one cares. No one is helping you. In fact, everyone seems against you. Weight loss is a path, which you have to walk alone, because only you can walk in your shoes. Only you can lose your weight.

There are plenty of support groups to help you. There are all sorts of help on the internet. I have friends on weight loss sites, which

I've had for years. Your church may have meetings to help. However, you are doing the work. You are walking the path to weight loss success or failure. Like going to church on Sunday, you receive encouragement and are now ready to tackle the world and then Monday comes along.

The encouragement has faded and now you face the prospect of another week with more challenges. You sense that alone feeling as you put an apple into your lunch bag and take it to work. Of course, in Christ, you are never alone, but when doing the weight loss journey, you may feel you are fighting the battle of the bulge all by yourself. You aren't. With Christ, you are more than enough to triumph over your excess weight. Though you have to walk out the weight loss journey in the flesh, you always have help in the spirit.

Excuse 145 - I Don't Have any Reason to Diet

If you have this excuse, you are pretty much without diet hope. No reason, no diet. Now if you aren't overweight, then good, but if you are overweight and say you can't find a good reason to diet, then you won't. Having a good reason for going on a weight loss diet is the catalyst for making it possible.

There are many reasons why you should diet. They are as individual as there are dieters. Obviously, the most common reason is just lose the weight. However, why do you want to lose weight? Most good reasons center on health. You want to lower blood pressure, for example. I watched my blood pressure go down each week as I lost weight. Maybe you want to lower triglycerides, or improve cholesterol. Perhaps you want to decrease heart disease risk. Then you might want to lower diabetes risk. Possibly, your joints hurt when walking. You huff and puff going up stairs. These are just a few of a whole slew of health reasons why you might want to lose weight. Better health or bad health prevention would be at the top of most people's reason list.

Here's a possible reason. "In the purchase of individual health insurance plans, weight is one of the factors that determines what the premium will be," says Susan Pisano, vice president of communications for America's Health Insurance Plans in Washington, D.C., an association representing health insurance companies. There is always the possibility a company could turn you down for health insurance. Overweight people are most likely to need the help with health costs.

Some people just want more energy. They want to play with their kids or grandkids. They want to be in a better mood, look better, and have an active lifestyle. Maybe in the process you can solve some personal issues that send you to the refrigerator. Without a good reason you will not have a successful weight loss journey.

Regardless of your diet method, you need a reason, as losing weight will be difficult at times. I call them the "mean times." Stop and ask yourself "why am I doing this." Just state your reason and keep on track.

Excuse 146 - I Don't Need To Diet

I hope this is true rather than an excuse. Going on a weight loss diet is a major step in life. If you don't need to diet, then don't. In fact, if you don't want to diet, then don't. We talk a great deal about weight loss, but we are only talking to overweight people. According to the National Institute of Diabetes and Digestive and Kidney Diseases, "More than two-thirds (68.8 percent) of adults are considered to be overweight or obese. More than one-third (35.7 percent) of adults are considered to be obese.

More than 1 in 20 (6.3 percent) have extreme obesity. Almost 3 in 4 men (74 percent) are considered to be overweight or obese." Therefore, there is 68.8 percent chance you are overweight. Now I don't want you to think you are overweight if you are not. You are not under condemnation.

"Our concern with people's weight needs to be thought about and spoken about by elders, not critics. We need the whole truth—that many women and girls suffer from this message (lose weight), many people don't need to lose weight, and that this message, simply put, does not help." David Bedrick, J.D., Dipl. PW.

While I believe overweight and obese people need to lose weight and being overweight is unhealthy, some want to minimize the call to diet. With them, I disagree. However, with them I agree there are those who don't need to diet but who think they should. Consider the following facts: 50-70% of normal-weight girls think they are overweight and 81% of 10-year-olds are afraid of being fat. The pressure for thinness is particularly acute in teenage girls. Going on diets to lose a little more weight, hating their looks, and wishing they looked better are symptoms of a society making looks relational to size. The message the country is growing more obese is true but the message everyone should be on a weight loss diet is not true. Since we should not listen to critics but us elders, diet only if you really need to. Get your identity not from the media but from Christ. Live life out in Christ.

On the other hand, there are plenty of online tools to decide if you really need to go on a diet. Your BMI (body mass index) is an indicator. The experts consider a **BMI of 24 or less a healthy weight**. Step on the scale and see how your weight matches some of the weight tables for your age and size. Look in the mirror checking for any bulges that don't belong there. You may be kidding yourself and need to lose those excess pounds. Don't diet if you don't need to, but start a weight loss diet if you need to lose some excess weight.

Excuse 147 – I Love Myself the Way I Am

That is a great first step. The Bible says to love others as you do yourself. That means you need to love yourself. In addition, know that God loves you just the way you are, even if you are overweight. Being in this place is one of most important things you can do for yourself.

But, (big but coming), if you really loved yourself, you would take care of yourself. We have established many times over that being overweight is unhealthy. Unhealthy means "harmful to your health." Loving yourself means doing no harm to yourself. Being overweight is definitely bringing potential harm to yourself. You are the only you in this world. If you really love yourself, you will make sure you cause no harm to come on you, just as you would your best friend. You are your "bestest" friend. True love cares.

Excuse 148 - Too Easy To Fall into Old Habits

I agree, certainly, when it comes to weight loss diets. They say you develop a new habit if you repeat an action for 28 days. Probably true for brushing your teeth, but with food the saying falls apart. You can go 30 days without eating a brownie, and on the 31st day someone hands you one, there goes your habit of not eating brownies. This is particularly true for us weight-challenged people. Skinny people might never eat a brownie.

Food habits are in a class all by themselves. When you go on a weight loss diet, you will have to make changes, a given. You will have to break old habits if you actually want to lose weight. You can't go into a diet thinking you will fall back into old eating habits once you reach your goal. You are just saying you will fail before you start. What you say has a great deal to do with what you do. Yes, we weight-loss challenged people easily fall back into old eating habits, but we aren't going to say we will, because our desire is to replace old habits with new good habits.

Always remember your present eating habits got you overweight. They are not good habits. They are the enemy to your health. You don't want to fall back into those old habits. The term is "fall" because falling is what going from eating well to eating poorly—the old habit cliff. Though falling is easy, get up and keep going. Lose the weight.

Excuse 149 – I Think I'm A Good Example of Just Being Myself.

I think you are saying you believe you are setting a good example to others, especially youth, of accepting yourself just as you are. I think people need to see models of people who accept themselves for who God created them to be. God created each of us unique and special. To portray that to others is important. Youth especially need to see they don't have to be like anyone else. They should be themselves.

The question we have to ask then is if you are overweight, what example does that show? Does it show it's okay to be fat when we all know it is so unhealthy? Does it show you don't care about yourself enough to take care of yourself? Maybe that example you think you are could be much better if you told others their health is important. Being overweight is not who you are. An example is what others see. What do people see about you?

Excuse 150 – I'm Not Perfect

Nobody is perfect when speaking of weight loss diets. Not exactly an excuse but just a statement of fact. However, some believe to go on a diet means following the plan perfectly in order to maximize the weight loss. The closer you stick to the plan you will have greater success in your weight loss journey.

However, we all know perfection isn't going to happen. In an ideal world and with an ideal diet plan, we could ideally stick to the diet perfectly.

Nothing, however, is ideal. Life happens. Schedules change. Stress and pressure occur. Life isn't perfect.

There are diets designed to play to that thought. There is the 90/10 and the 80/20 diet plans because they already know you aren't going to be perfect. Their thought is if you are 80% or 90%

good then you will still reach your goals and not be so frustrated. Some diets even have cheat days, because everyone knows you aren't going to be perfect and will get frustrated in trying. I don't think we should go into the process planning not to stick to our diet plan.

I've found in my dieting when I make an intentional slipup it puts me on a slippery slope to bingeing. I don't think we should approach dieting with the idea we're going to cheat. We might, but we didn't plan to cheat. I think you should try for maximum progress and if you slip up occasionally, just move on. No shame, no condemnation. Yes, none of us is perfect in our weight loss journey. Accept the fact and just do it.

Excuse 151 – It's Inner Beauty That Really Matters

If you are an overweight women you may have heard someone say, "you have such a pretty face." At first, you felt good about the compliment until you realize that they are saying your face is pretty, but the rest of you is not. Your resulting comeback might be that inner beauty is what really matters.

People say that inner beauty is something ugly people say to themselves to feel better. Inner beauty by definition is something experienced in a person's character that brings beauty to the world. Are you bringing something pretty to the world? Is it a servant's heart, a humble attitude, or even a positive attitude?

True beauty is different for everyone, but must reflect something good, honest, and kind, just to mention a few things. When I was at a ministry conference, the leader told the people on the stage to dress up. The thought was even though God doesn't look at the outer appearance, people do, and what they see reflects on both themselves and the organization.

The ideal is inner beauty wrapped in a healthy looking package. People can see your inner beauty easier when they see you take care of yourself.

Excuse 152 – It's A Bad Time to Diet

For most people, the time of the year is a bad time to start a diet. They may be off work, going on a trip over the New Years, and still finishing the Christmas cookies. Therefore, Christmas is a bad time to start. How about New Years? How about during vacation time in the summer? When you really get down to the bottom line, is there a good time to diet? In most lives, busyness is going on all the time. Weight loss diet would just add to all the stuff.

Is there really a bad time to diet? Would postponing weight loss really make you healthier? Delay is the key to failure. You have to eat every day, why don't you just eat on a weight loss diet. Simple enough. Just change your diet a little. Yes, everyone is on a diet. What we eat is a diet. Cows eat a diet of grass. Some diets are weight loss diets, some weight gain. Just change your diet a little and lose weight in the process. Today is never a bad time to get on the weight loss journey.

Excuse 153 - I'll Start Tomorrow

Procrastination is a blight no dieter should dare to endure. Saying you are putting off your weight loss journey is just saying you aren't going to diet. Did you know there is no tomorrow? Tomorrow never comes. Tomorrow is always tomorrow. Today is not tomorrow.

Putting dieting off to a more convenient time is saying I'm not going to diet. There are no convenient times. Charlene and I go on a trip almost every month, and if we waited until we weren't traveling, we would never reach our goal. If you blow your diet each weekend and start your diet every Monday morning, you are not dieting. There has to be weight loss in a weight loss diet or else you aren't on a weight loss diet.

I'll start tomorrow. That just reminds me of Annie's song *Tomorrow*. "it's always a day away!" What do they say: tomorrow never comes? Or like Mark Twain: "Never *put off* till *tomorrow* what may be done day after *tomorrow* just as well." Or as some say, "why do today what you can put off until tomorrow."

We are not promised a tomorrow. We have today. If you want to see change in your life, you have to start today. Benjamin Franklin said the famous quote—"Don't *put off* until *tomorrow* what you can do today." When it comes to weight and health, **today** is the best day to begin. Don't slip doing something to tomorrow, and then let it slide to the next day, and the next.

Procrastination is the path to failure. Even the Bible says, "Don't put it off; do it now! Don't rest until you do" (Proverbs 6:4). Alternatively, as the Nike slogan goes, "Just do it." Successful people manage their time. If something needs done, they take action immediately. If you need to lose weight, begin now.

I'll certainly be the first to admit dieting can be a struggle. Fat reduction is all about **why** you are dieting and about whom you lean on for help. So don't let another year go by without meeting your goal. This time next year, you could be at your goal if you start today. Like pigs, excuses don't fly.

<u>Excuse 154 – If ...</u>

No ifs, ands, or buts. The phrase is over 150 years old, and used in various works during the 1800s. For instance, *New York Daily Times* newspaper wrote in the year 1854, *"No ifs or ands or buts about it."* How about the saying, "If ifs, ands, and buts were candies and nuts we'd all have a merry Christmas."

One issue I've personally observed from following different diets is the questions people have about the diet. Yes, there are legitimate questions like what I can substitute for fish (I hate fish). However, there are always those who add the "ifs, ands, or buts." I don't like fish so can I substitute chocolate. From these three words excuses come slipping out of our mouths. Would you be okay **<u>if</u>** I start next Month? Can I have coffee **<u>and</u>** cream? **<u>But</u>** I can't do pushups.

Excuses and reasons for not doing things are easy to use. Stick to the plan without excuses or doubts. When they take away from your success, they mean failure. If they add to your success by clarification, they are good. The chances they are bad are greater than they are good. Therefore, no "ifs, ands, or buts."

Excuse 155 - I Just Don't Want to Diet

This is perhaps the most honest excuse of them all. I don't know anyone who wants to go on a weight loss diet. Change is hard. You must have courage to change from the familiar to the new. George Bernard Shaw said, "Progress is impossible without change, and those who cannot change their minds cannot change anything."

If you are overweight, then you need to lose weight. However, if you don't want to and ultimately don't lose weight, you live with the results. My suggestion is if you don't want to lose weight, have a good reason you don't lose weight. Just as you need a good reason to lose weight, you need a good reason you won't lose weight.

If you don't like where you are with your weight, then only you can change the situation. Robin Sharma said, "Change is hard at first, messy in the middle, and gorgeous at the end." Nothing happens in life until you make a change. Don't diet if you don't want to diet, because dieting takes commitment and resolution to walk through a weight-loss journey. If you just don't want to go through the weight loss process, it's entirely your decision. Weight loss is not always easy. I know because I walk the weight loss path every day.

Chapter 5

Event Excuses

I call this section event excuses because they revolve around certain events that occur in our lives which might be cause for weight loss problems. Even though these events might occur once a year, if you add them all up, you face many days of possible weight loss challenges. An excuse is an excuse whether about your birthday or ground hog day.

Excuse 156 – It's Wednesday

Or Friday, or a day of the week ending in "day." What day of the week is your weakest day for dieting? If you work, you will probably say Friday. The workweek is over and you just want to let down your guard and let loose a little. Maybe your fellow workers went out to lunch on Friday. Friday for us was often pizza night. Maybe you have a meeting on a particular night of the week.

An excuse isn't limited to time such as a day of the week. Excuses can pop out of our mouths anytime. Some days do pose as problematic, but for the weight loss dieter, all days are created equal, some are just more challenging. Remember solutions over excuses. Take every day at a time and solve the issues of the now. Don't look to tomorrow for problems only planning.

Excuse 157 – It's Valentine's Day

February 14 is Valentine's Day, both a fact, and an excuse. Valentine's Day is the fourth holiday behind Christmas, Halloween, and Easter for the most candy sold. I think the little candies with the one or two words on them are one of the first candies I remember as a child. Candy companies still make them. In fact, they invented the process for cutting the Sweethearts candies in 1847 and they stamped the words on them starting in 1866. I also like those little red hots with the powerful cinnamon kick making your tongue red. They came out in the 1930's. Enough reminiscing. Eating all the candy started me on my love for candy. Now candy is just so much sugar.

I guess what I'm saying is don't let a special occasion get out of hand. You don't need any of the candy. Maybe a nice dinner out on plan. You don't need another excuse to go off your weight loss diet. Valentine's Day says love and should be the norm for every day. Stay the weight loss road and don't let Valentine's Day get you sidetracked. Life may be like a box of chocolates, just don't eat the box.

Excuse 158- It's My Birthday

Not mine, at least not until July, but birthdays are another day where you might be tempted to overdo and sidetrack your diet. There is no song called "It's my birthday and I'll overeat if I want to." I know birthdays only come once a year and so does every holiday, family, and relative's birthday, and office Christmas party. Once a year is a quick way to sabotage your whole weight loss journey.

Okay, a birthday is another milestone in your life, and a cause of celebration and a great time to thank God for another year of life. There are ways to celebrate without overeating. Maybe go out to a dinner at a place you like and stay on plan—maybe a small steak, asparagus or other vegetable, ½ baked potato, and small side salad. Leave off the toppings and just enjoy the day. You might be able to have a bite or two of cake. I find the problem with any indulging is the slippery slope you might end up on to diet disaster. I have personally found eating a bite of cake, for example, lowers my guard, and I eat the whole piece of cake. Maybe I don't gain, maybe I do a little, but the extra bites throw off my diet for a few days. Be careful what you eat, even if on your birthday.

Excuse 159 – It's A Holiday

"Today is a holiday." Much like your birthday, a holiday only comes once a year. "But wait"…as the infomercial always adds. There are 10 federal holidays. There are bunches of religious holidays, commonly celebrated days—such as Mother's Day, Father's Day, election day, state holidays—such as Mardi Gras, school holidays, and business holidays—such as day after Thanksgiving. So wait just a minute. If you went off your diet on every possible holiday, you wouldn't be on your diet much.

However, you still can celebrate holidays. You might celebrate July 4 with a BBQ, but stick to the plan. You can take mom out to lunch on Mother's Day, but go where you can stay on plan. What about all those national whatchamacallit days, such as chocolate day, donut day, or taco day? Ignore them. You don't need any more distractions to make your diet impossible. There are plenty of ways to celebrate and remain on track. Don't let the day, whatever you call it, be a reason to miss getting your weight off.

Excuse 160 – It's Vacation Tomorrow

Maybe you're starting vacation tomorrow or next week. As a retired senior, we don't go on vacation we go on trips. A vacation is "a period of suspension of work, study, or other activity, usually used for rest, recreation, or travel." Other than the actual travel, our travel days are pretty much the same as usual. The time getting ready for a trip can be a time to let down your guard, go out to eat, or just begin the vacation eating.

Vacations or trips require planning. If you aren't a planner, then you're in deep difficultly. If you are a spontaneous type, trips or vacations will be more difficult while on a weight loss diet. There have been times we just let go and gained 10-to-15 pounds on a long trip. Pounds are easy to put on but hard to take off. Instead of thinking you are taking a vacation from your diet, take your diet on vacation with you. Okay have a treat, but get in some walking or hiking. Don't delay your diet because of a trip. Learn to manage your weight loss journey while on vacation. If you eat out more, then eat according to plan. It's all good.

Excuse 161 - We Go Camping Every Weekend

I'm not sure what you mean by "camping." I like to camp out in a motel room. Others take their RV to the woods to camp. Many years ago, I was a Scoutmaster, and we hiked into our campsite with only what we could carry. I call sleeping in a pup tent real roughing it camping. We also had tailgate camping, which was driving to the campsite and setting up our tents.

The word "camping" means something different to everyone. The dictionary defines camping as, "the activity spending a vacation living in a camp, tent, or camper." So what does all this have to do with weight loss? Not much. You have to eat wherever you go. Therefore, you stay on your weight loss plan wherever you go. Whether you're roughing it or camping in a large RV, you still eat according to plan. Sorry you can't use this as an excuse. In fact, on the little camping I've done, eating less was normal. We didn't sit around and watch TV. There is activity going on. Maybe boating, hiking, exploring, and other physical activities go along with camping. So go camping every weekend and take your weight loss plan with you.

No S'mores for you.

Excuse 162 - But It's the Weekend

This is a big excuse for people who work. I remember working all week, sticking to the plan, and when the weekend came, I regained all I had lost. This went from week to week. Going out to eat on the weekend. Dropping the guard and dropping the weight loss plan over the weekend, with an "I'll get back on track on Monday." Folks, weekday only dieting doesn't work. You never make progress and often gain instead of lose. Weight loss is easier for me now since I'm retired and every day is pretty much the same as any other day. People who look to the weekend to go off their diet will not succeed at a weight loss journey.

Weight loss has to be a day-by-day matter. Monday, Tuesday...Saturday, and Sunday. Cheat days don't work, and especially weekend cheat days. A cheat day only allows you to cheat yourself. If you have been on a diet long, you will quickly discover the difficulty in taking a pound off but how easy for you to put one on. We work all week to get two pounds off, by following the plan to the tee, only to gain two or three pounds back over the weekend. No progress. Cross weekends off your calendar.

Excuse 163 - Too Many Events Coming Up

When we drive out to California, usually in April and May, weight loss is very challenging. This could easily have been our excuse. In fact, very problematic. Most of us have lots going on in our lives. Some have a busy social calendar. We think these events will interfere with going on a weight loss diet. Well, they do present challenges, no doubt, but this is going to happen regardless of whether you go on a diet or not. If you postpone your diet, you just keep adding to the weight problem. To add the cherry to the sundae these events will also add to your weight problem, if you don't have a plan.

When we travel, we have a travel diet plan. Yes, the plan doesn't always work out, but the trip goes better for us than if we have no plan. Most events involve eating. Birthdays, holidays, church functions, and meeting friends normally have the component of food. Time for your plan to kick in. You develop a strategy for eating during these events. Cut me the smallest piece of birthday cake and I'll split the piece with my wife. There are plenty of ways to maintain a weight loss diet and still enjoy the events. No excuses, please.

Excuse 164 - I Travel Too Much

I will be the first to admit travel can take a toll on dieting. To keep on track requires a great deal more planning. When you travel on business, situations you didn't plan for will confront you. I know when I went to Sao Paulo on business they had planned places for us to eat. Brazil steakhouse one night, an all-you-can eat steak place. Therefore, travel is a problem. A few people are traveling weekly. You might even travel somewhere and stay for several weeks on a project. I find traveling for your company especially hard because the company is paying the bill and you are getting to try new foods. Actual and reasonable.

I went to a meeting recently to hear a speaker talk about his weight loss journey since he had reached his goal. His big problem was company travel. When they met, there was always big layouts of food and unlimited drinks. He simply overate and gained weight. He had to overcome this one problem if he was to lose. He decided weight loss and health was more important so ate foods on plan and small portions. He also took a small cold food bag to work with what he could eat. He worked on the diet each time he traveled and he reached his goal. His health markers really improved.

You will find a way to eat those meals in proper portions and still lose weight. You have to decide the importance you have on losing weight. We travel about one week a month, which means trying times for maintaining our weight. In some cases, we just want to break even. Might mean doing some extra walking. You can do it, though, especially if you really want to lose the weight. You might have to take your snacks with you. You will have to think outside of the box and will require some self-control. Search on dieting while travelling for tips.

You need a new mindset when you need to lose weight. Losing weight becomes important and you find ways to accomplish the task no matter what the obstacles. Traveling just adds to the obstacles, but there are still solutions to every difficulty.

Chapter 6

Emotional Excuses

We come up with these excuses when life has us emotionally stretched. Stress, mental tiredness, and just poor thinking can ruin a weight loss diet. Look at these excuses and see if any resonate in your brain.

Excuse 165 - I Love Food

I think this is one of the most common excuses and one of the most difficult to overcome. In his book, *If My Body Is a Temple, Then I Was a Megachurch,* Scott Davis in his struggles with obesity concluded he just loved food. I was just about to say I know of no one who hates food, but doing a search reveals there are some who actually hate food. However, they have a whole set of different problems.

Most of us weight challenged folk love to eat. I love to go to church potlucks and try out different pots of food. I like a chili cook-off where I can try new chili styles. I love the dessert bar at Golden Corral or Ryan's. I love Italian, Mexican, Chinese, comfort foods, fast food, and the Jewish deli. For those of us who are trying to stay on a diet—big problem.

When I drive out of my subdivision and head for the freeway, there are at least two dozen eateries all tugging at my genuine love for food. However, I have to stifle the thought if I'm going to lose weight. I can substitute some of those foods in a more calorie friendly way and help my cause. However, those places will always be looming in the background ready to pounce.

Loving food means we have to take some crucial steps to make weight loss a possibility. We have to love to eat the food we have to eat in order to lose weight. We have to eat food with exciting flavors and varieties to help us love the food we need to eat and still lose weight. Some would say that is an unacceptable sacrifice, but what is carrying all the extra weight doing to you. Are you carrying around a 50-pound bag of rocks each day, maybe even a hundred? Some people can't even lift 50 pounds but they are needlessly hauling the extra weight around on their body every step they take. Loving food is never going away, so love the food you have to eat.

Excuse 166 – I'm Too Tired

How can you say you're too tired to diet? Dieting is just eating. Now, if you're saying you're too tired to go to the gym and work out, okay I get you. Many people go work out in the morning before the day begins. With these 24-hour gyms, you can go anytime and work out. I don't go to a gym. I walk. Since I walk during the day or in the morning, I'm usually not too tired. There is a way or an excuse.

Another problem especially in the evening, being tired can lower your defenses to temptation. When this happens to me, I get an "I don't care attitude" and a bad attitude isn't good. I'll say I'm going to fix me a peanut butter sandwich. Charlene will ask do you really need the sandwich. No I don't. You really have to be on guard when you're tired. A good reason why getting a good night's sleep is so important.

Being overweight adds to the tiredness. There was a time I never missed my afternoon nap. Now I've lost weight, I infrequently take a nap. You just naturally have more energy when you are not carrying around all the extra poundage. I was carrying around a backpack filled with 50 pounds of baloney. If you are overweight, no wonder you are always weary. Get the weight off and get your energy back.

Excuse 167 – I'm Too Overweight

I'm not sure how to answer this one. You're too overweight to diet. Hmmm. Isn't the whole purpose of dieting, to lose the weight? If you have watched the program *My 600 Pound Life,* you will see people too heavy to move. However, they have to diet to lose the weight. Unfortunately, some don't live long enough to lose the weight. Weight in extreme excess is enormously burdensome and dangerous on the critical functions of the body.

People over 500 pounds diet. I know many who had to take the surgery path to weight loss because of issues they had with dieting. However, not issues because they were overweight, but issues which made them overweight. At such weight, they are morbidly obese. Therefore, not too overweight to diet. In fact, they must diet to get the weight down.

However, what I really hear is I'm too overweight to exercise. Anytime you are very overweight you always need to get your healthcare provider's okay to exercise. You may need to get some weight off simply dieting first. On the other hand, you may start very slowly, walking a little. You might do some exercises while seated. Check the internet for types of exercises you can do while seated. There is a solution for every excuse.

If your excuse is stronger than your desire to overcome, then you will simply be one of the 95% who don't lose weight—another negative statistic. However, you can reach your goal no matter your weight, and reducing will help your joints walk you wherever you would like to go. How about walk on the beach, or hike a trail through the mountains. This is a no excuse.

<u>Excuse 168 – I'm Feeling Sorry for Myself</u>

Sounds pathetic when you think about this excuse. Sitting on the couch feeling sorry for yourself because you are overweight. That just isn't going to help the situation. I don't know your circumstances, or how you got to your state of obesity, but many have had some traumatic event triggering the weight gain. The event happened in the past. However, you can't live in the past. You have to pick up and move on, for your sake and those around you. You have to take care of yourself to find both physical and mental strength to help others.

You may need some professional counseling. Maybe you need to talk with someone who can help you get past the trauma and move on.

I'm hoping you are not so in-ward looking you can't see there are many people who need you. When you think poor me, you don't see how negatively your life affects others.

You might say I have no one who cares for me. Then now is the time to get out there and help people. Volunteer somewhere and show you care for others and soon people will care about you. You are important and others need your help.

I know some days don't go so well. Maybe you even think life is picking on you. Maybe you even think God is picking on you. Totally not true. Don't believe the lie. No one is picking on you but your mind. Get up off the couch and fix you some tea. Relax and see everything is going to be okay.

<u>Excuse 169 - I Deserve A Break</u>

"You deserve a break today." I'm sure you've heard the slogan by McDonalds. I also saw the same idea in a Publix commercial as a woman stood in front of the dessert counter—"you deserve it"—she thought. Luxury cars promote you deserve the luxury and comfort of their car. Businesses use the idea all the time and to get in our heads, so there's no wonder we will come up with an excuse to take a break from dieting, whether a meal, a day or a week. I know I have similar thoughts from time to time.

Hey, I did very well this week, and I deserve a brownie. Deserve means, "to have earned something or be given something because of your actions or qualities." We get the idea we earned a break because of all our good dieting this week. However, you haven't done any more than you should have done in order to get your weight off. What you earned is the weight loss. You worked hard to get a pound off, so you don't want to take a break and put 5 pounds back on.

You don't need to have a setback because you went off your plan to give yourself a break. You deserve to lose weight. You deserve the health you gain from losing the weight. You deserve to be trim and fit. You don't deserve a sugary food delaying you from reaching your goals. So don't let this excuse escape your lips and end up on your hips.

Excuse 170 – I'm Bored

"I'm bored" is a familiar excuse. I hear the excuse coming from my head quite often. I spend a great deal of time writing, and sometimes I just get bored sitting all day. I saw this cartoon recently. "There are **2 reasons I'm fat. I eat when I'm bored and I'm always bored.**"

The Cambridge Dictionary says bored means, "feeling tired and unhappy because something is not interesting or because you have nothing to do." Wikipedia defines bored as, "an emotional or psychological state experienced when an individual is left without anything in particular to do, is not interested in his or her surroundings, or feels that a day or period is dull or tedious." I think most people feel bored at times. Some might feel bored, but they get up and do something about the boredom. The worst case is boredom leads to despairing of life.

You can even be bored when you are busy, even though keeping busy is usually the answer to being bored. I find I need to vary my busy-ness. After writing for a long time, I'll find something else to do. Watching TV doesn't usually help with boredom just the opposite. We do have a few programs we enjoy on TV and will watch and relax from the daily writing.

Being bored while on a weight loss journey is a serious matter. I feel bored at times and my first instinct is to get up and eat something. Well, eating is certainly not going to help a weight loss diet. I know seniors who have the problem just because they have nothing to do, at least think they have nothing to do. You have to fight boredom in order to have success on the weight loss journey. Make a list of items you need to do, and add to the list items you want to do, somewhat as a bucket list. Think big. I use to have a list of 100 things I wanted to accomplish in the year. Amazing how many you finish and check off when you have a list. Some were big such as hiking to Mt. LeConte and stay in the lodge for three nights, which we did. Others to read the top best sellers list and Oprah's list.

However, this isn't an excuse to go off your weight loss journey. Sometimes I just get a glass of water. Other times I cheat. If you are bored with your diet plan, now there is a completely different matter. If you are, you probably won't stick to the plan. So try varying the fruits and veggies you can have. Try new recipes. Experiment with seasonings. Surf restaurant menus to see what they have that fits your plan. Vary the menu from lunch to dinner. Maybe even reverse your meals and eat eggs for dinner, etc. Fight the bored feeling by looking at the prize and pressing for the goal.

Excuse 171 – It's Been a Bad Day

We all have some of those days, which try men's souls. Maybe a flat tire, maybe the washing machine goes on the fritz, or maybe an unpleasant confrontation at work. Many factors might trigger you to think today was a bad day. Perhaps you had a relationship problem, so you feel like tossing the diet out the window and getting into a bag of chips or a gallon of ice cream. There might be a little comfort in ice cream, but nothing you can eat really can change what went on in your day. This excuse can get you off track and off your diet.

So beware of bad days. Which means you have to change your thinking about what is bad. This goes beyond just dieting. This involves how you handle adversity in life. Do you let difficulties rule your life? On the other hand, do you put them in their place? You can choose. I know choosing is not always easy, but some people begin to have bad days every day—the bad day habit. Then you almost expect to have bad days or worse yet even, want them. Don't let bad days be normal, and don't let them win over your weight loss journey. You have the power to overcome.

Excuse 172 – I'm In a Bad Mood

This opens up the whole area of emotional eating. If you are sitting on the couch in the evening in a bad mood, you are unleashing the dynamics of dieting disaster. The dreaded binge eating trying to make your bad mood good. As Dr. Phil would say, "how's that working for you?" Crystal Gayle sang a song called "Don't It Make My Brown Eyes Blue." I always sing that phrase as "donuts make my brown eyes blue." As if, food can change mood.

Food on bad days may give you something to do—to control. You are probably in a bad mood because something went wrong during the day. You felt you lost control of your life. One detail you can control is eating for better or worse.

Are you really in control if you sit and eat all evening? You are just adding to the guilt you feel because you wasted a day by going off the weight loss plan. Sometimes those days turn into weeks if you don't handle the issue that turned your good mood into bad. In some way, you have to look at why you are in this bad mood. Is this what your life has become, and what can you do to reverse the direction you are going now. This isn't just about dieting. This is about how you handle difficult days. Learn to handle them and every area of your life will improve. Don't let your mood govern your life. Stick to the plan and make your life better.

Excuse 173 – I'm Too Stressed

Stress is unpleasant. Extreme stress is miserable. Stress affects all areas of your life and not just weight loss. Experts have linked numerous emotional and physical disorders to stress. If you look up symptoms of stress on the internet, you will see tons of them. However, what we are looking at is the excuse you can't go on a weight loss diet or can't maintain one because you say, "I'm too stressed."

You have to eat whether stressed or not so why not just eat what's on your plan. I know, not so easy, as we are used to having some comforting foods to help us cope. Mom always fixed a bowl of ice cream so I want ice cream. You might want a box of cookies or crackers. Whatever is your food of choice for relieving the stress you won't be going for the carrot sticks. These are the times that try man's diet.

I'm going to take this excuse as if you mean life has you really stressed. First, you need to identify the sources of your stress. Is your stress factor work, relationships, finances, other activities? You need to write down what you think are stress factors. Is the stress causing you to eat more than you should? Do you sit in front of the TV at night and snack?

Second, look at the list and you will probably notice you have little control over the sources of stress. Your boss is too demanding for example. You need the job, maybe even love the job, but you think the boss is your stress. You can't control the boss, so how are you going to handle the problem.

Turn it over to the Lord, and rest in Him. Don't let this stuff control your life. Enjoy your life as God designed stress free living. Don't let stress get to you. Nip it in the bud.

Excuse 174 - I Get No Support

If you are looking for support, you must be looking in the wrong places. Okay, you may not get much support from your family, especially if they are all fat or if your spouse doesn't want to diet or doesn't need to diet. Your kids are little help as they are always demanding your time and clamoring for sugary foods you don't want to give them.

First, you must have the mindset you are in this for yourself. You have a life and you should have a say in how it goes. You can't care what anyone thinks. You know you have to lose weight, to resolve health issues, or prevent them. You are willing to do whatever you have to do to reach your goals. You may have to make two different meals. You may have to buy foods for your family you can't have. You may be able to sneak in a few healthy meals in the process.

Second, no one can help you anyway. You are in this for yourself. I say no one can help you in the sense you are the one who puts the spoon to your mouth. I'm always concerned, however, when family doesn't want to help in losing the weight. A real relationship means helping one another. The husband and wife are helpmates rendering assistance when needed.

Third, you can get a lot of encouragement from various websites. There are many forums about any diet subject. Whether you are struggling with emotional eating, or need help on your plan, there is help available. I've had friends on SparkPeople, for example, for years.

You aren't alone in this journey. If there's no support at home, reach out and find your niche. Plus. God is always at your side ready to help. Lean on Him when you feel alone in this weight loss journey.

Excuse 175 – I'm Too Lazy

Maybe, but you can still follow a simple weight loss plan. There are generally two parts to a weight loss plan—diet and exercise. Now I'm sure you are not too lazy to eat or else you wouldn't be overweight. Unless you mean you are too lazy to fix your food and you just go get fast food. Then Houston we have a problem.

Most experts consider diet 80-90% of weight loss. Therefore, diet is the most important part of losing weight. You might find some fitness trainers saying the more exercise the better. If we are talking weight loss then you can lose weight without exercise, if you are too lazy to exercise.

Unfortunately, people profile heavy people as being lazy. In fact, if you are lazy, then you might be overweight. I don't want the lazy label and I'm sure you don't want that label either. Don't be lazy. There is a life to live and enjoy. There is plenty of medical evidence stating a healthy diet and exercise will improve and maintain your quality of life. This excuse is not flattering in any way, shape, or form. Get off the couch and fix your food so you can get out there and walk and enjoy life. Change lazy into more active. Hey, it's your only life here. Make it the best possible life you can.

Excuse 176- I'm Too Upset

This is in the category of emotional eating. The dictionary says the word upset means, "a state of being unhappy, disappointed, or worried." The excuse usually comes when you say phooey on the plan and grab a bag of chips. Maybe your upset food is ice cream or cupcakes. Whatever the food is, it usually isn't celery sticks. Stuff happens in life when we least expect it, and can be very upsetting. If you have kids, you get upset often. What did she or he do now?

I'm not sure what you mean by "too" upset. Sounds like the last straw upset. You will have to face this obstacle. If you're on a weight-loss diet, you have to face the problem head-on and don't let it ruin your hard work. Don't use food to salve the hurt or disappointment. Take a few deep breaths and know this too will pass.

Take care of yourself. Go for a walk or take a nice bath. Remember there are always alternate ways to deal with emotions than eating or even not eating. Know you are never alone in these situations and there is always a way out. Don't become depressed. Count it all joy. Cast the care on the Lord.

Chapter 7

Medical Excuses

These are not necessarily excuses, but real situations in your health. They become an excuse when they prevent you from losing weight. Weight itself is the cause of many health problems so removing the issues will help in the overall medical situations plaguing you. I could have lumped the excuses into one excuse, but several we hear all the time, and we can discuss them individually. Again, if you have any of these health-related excuses and are under a doctor's care, follow his or her instructions.

Excuse 177 - I Have a Bad Knee

An excuse but also a fact. When we speak of any physical limitation, you might have to adjust the exercise part of weight loss. You might have a bad knee, a bad shoulder, a bad neck, a bad back, whatever limits physical movement or is painful.

First, remember exercise is a small percentage of weight loss. Nothing about a bad knee can keep you from sticking to your eating plan. Any body part giving you pain when standing such as the knee, hip, ankle, etc. you should avoid exercises causing those parts pain. Avoid impact exercises like running or sports having fast changes of direction, but you can still perform weight loss exercises with a high degree of intensity.

Do a search for exercises to do with your bad knee. If your knee is very bad, you might not be able to stand, so sitting could work. You are probably under a physician's care at this point. What I'm saying here is physical limitations could be an excuse to not lose weight but don't let excuses set you up for failure. In fact, getting the weight off will probably help those bad joints. God did not design your joints to carry an extra 50 to 100 pounds or more. Stick with the eating plan, and do what you can do with your limitation. No excuses, please.

Excuse 178 - I'm Allergic to...

You might consider this a reason not to eat certain foods, but not an excuse for weight loss dieting. The percentage of food allergies are climbing every year. Researchers estimate 15 million people in the US have food allergies. Sounds a lot but only 4% of the people living here. Now many add into the mix sensitivities to foods such as dairy, soy, wheat, etc. People with allergies have to be careful what they eat. Some allergic reactions can lead to serious problems, even death, so they are factors you should consider carefully when going on a weight loss diet.

However, the weight loss diet is still possible. After all, you still have to eat. I did see a young boy on TV who is allergic to almost everything, definitely an extreme allergy problem. Most people with allergies have one or two types of food they are allergic to such as nuts, shellfish, etc. Just leave the suspect item off the diet if your plan lists those foods to eat on the diet. Simply avoid the food to which you are allergic. You might want to get a food sensitivity check to see what other foods you might want to avoid. Many people are sensitive to soy for example. Soy is in many foods. Charlene had many problems with a diet that included various products with soy. She had to stop eating those, but continued on the diet plan and lost weight. So check the ingredients before eating. Keep on the plan and lose the weight.

Excuse 179 - Dieting Makes Me Constipated

This can be a problem especially if you are on a low-carb diet. If you have cut out whole grains or wheat, you may have a tendency to go slow. Chronic constipation is infrequent bowel movements or difficult passage of stools persisting for several weeks or longer. The medical community describes constipation as having fewer than three bowel movements a week. Yikes. High protein diets tend to have less fruit and vegetables. Harder to get the needed fiber when you cut back on veggies.

Try to get in some high fiber veggies along with fruits. I know most low-carb diets don't add much fruit. Some diets eliminate fruit. If your diet allows, eat more beans. Make sure you drink **lots** of water. Maybe cut or eliminate the caffeine as it might act as a diuretic and take water from the digestion track. Cut your stress if possible. A natural laxative could help. We get a tea called *Smooth Move,* which helps with occasional problems. In the end if diet causes a serious condition for you, consider doing a different diet. Constipation is annoying to say the least, but dangerous to say the worse. Still there are ways around the problems. No excuses.

Excuse 180 - I Have Diabetes

We are talking about type two diabetes or pre-diabetes. Eighty five percent of diabetics are overweight. "HSPH's Willett, who chairs the Department of Nutrition, said that getting Americans' diet right can mean the difference between being healthy or ill. Studies have shown that not smoking, eating properly, and keeping a healthy weight—a body mass index of under 25—reduces the risk of diabetes by 90 percent. Apart from lung cancer, there is no other disease that can be almost eliminated with simple lifestyle changes"

This is a conundrum. You don't want to go on a weight loss diet because you have diabetes, but there is an 85% chance you have diabetes because you are overweight and a 90% chance you can get rid of the issue by losing the weight.

Studies have shown losing just 7 percent of one's body weight can increase insulin sensitivity 57 percent. Diabetes is a disease where you lose insulin sensitivity. Therefore, I would think if you have diabetes or pre-diabetes, the first step you would want to take is get your weight under control. As with any diagnosed problem, you need to follow your doctor's orders. You will need a diet appropriate for the diabetic. There is plenty of help on the web. Your doctor may put you together with a nutritionist who will set your diet plan. You have a good chance of getting rid of this problem through diet and lose the weight.

Excuse 181 - I Have a Hormone Problem

Hormones are your body's chemical messengers. They help control practically every physiological process in your body. A precise hormonal balance is vital to proper body functioning. Certain foods in your diet can restore or throw off the balance of your hormones. Eating a well-balanced diet is essential. The fact you can say you have a hormone problem is half the battle. If true, a proper diet could restore your hormone problems. Your doctor can help if you need medical assistance to repair the wayward hormones. Follow your doctor's advice and take the needed prescriptions. There is always a possibility of serious problems with some of the body's hormone makers.

For women, hormones play an even bigger role in well-being. Some of the foods you may have to avoid are red meat, sugar, some fruits, caffeine, grains, especially wheat, dairy, and then go through a detoxification process. There is plenty of help on the web. I just looked at Maria Shriver's website and there is much help there.

There are at least three main hormones that help in weight loss—leptin, cortisol, and ghrelin. These hormones you'll want to keep in shape if you are trying to lose weight. You can learn about them by looking them up on the web.

You need to reset the hormone imbalances, and they are probably "out of whack" because of your diet. Get a weight loss diet started to help those hormones. Just 21 days could get you back on track. It's no excuse especially if a good diet will restore those hormones.

Excuse 182 - I Suffer From Insomnia

Roughly, 60 million Americans suffer from insomnia. Watch TV commercials and many will be about sleep aids. Insomnia causes daytime tiredness and lack of sleep can lead to a higher risk of chronic health problems like high blood pressure, heart disease, and stroke. In addition, evidence links lack of quality sleep to increased risk of obesity. Sounds like a catch 22. Missing sleep creates a vicious cycle in your body, making you more prone to various factors contributing to weight gain. If you're overweight and suffer from insomnia, you are at risk for additional health problem including sleep apnea. Therefore, of first importance get the weight off.

Weight loss is a detail you can do now, which in itself might cure the insomnia. Of course, there are many reasons why a person can't sleep—stress, worry, depression, anger, grief, and many emotional conditions. If you tried weight loss dieting, and it only added to your stress and anxiety, the diet could have been the problem. Too much restriction can cause anxiety, as well as an unhealthy diet with too much sugar for example can cause problems. Eliminate the conditions causing weight gain, and then weight loss will be easier.

Excuse 183 - I Have a Slow Metabolism

If you're overweight, slow metabolism may be just the opposite according to the Mayo Clinic. They say slow metabolism is rare. Metabolism is the process by which your body converts what you eat and drink into energy. Your metabolism is pretty much set for your system but you can impair the process by a number of factors. Getting no exercise will slow down the process your body uses to burn energy. As you get older, the amount of energy used is less so appears like a slowdown in metabolism. Eating too much, exercising too little, and certain medical conditions can slow down the metabolism.

However, you look at it; your metabolism isn't a valid excuse for not losing weight. You can't speed up energy burning while sitting on the couch eating Twinkies. Don't worry about your metabolism unless your doctor says you have a specific problem. Then don't worry anyway. Find a plan and stay on track. Get plenty of both aerobic and strength exercise. Keep fit as they say, and keep working on the weight loss diet. Your metabolism will take care of itself.

Excuse 184 - I'm On Medication

Not exactly an excuse, but a fact, if indeed you mean doctor authorized medication. Some people call a bottle of vodka medication. Maybe you can remember the Baldwin sisters on the TV series "The Waltons" who made an elixir using a special recipe. If you really are on official medications then this doesn't negate a weight loss diet, but may need further scrutiny. Some medications conflict with certain foods, such as grapefruit. You have to take into account what medication you are taking and if there are any foods, which you must avoid. Then pick a weight loss diet without those foods and stick to the plan. If you are taking diabetes, high blood pressure, or obesity related drugs, then good news. Losing weight may very well lower or eliminate your need for these drugs.

Any condition caused by obesity or being overweight will most likely go away when you aren't obese or overweight. Just don't let your obesity go to the point you damage your health. Joint pain can become joint replacement because of weight. Heart disease might have damaged the heart. The bottom line is to get the weight off first. As always, check with your doctor before changing or reducing any medication. Eating healthy goes a long way to keeping healthy.

Excuse 185 - I Have a Thyroid Problem

There are all kinds of thyroid problems, including the removal of the thyroid. Each problem has its own therapy and medical prognosis. According to Wikipedia, "the thyroid gland or simply the thyroid is an endocrine gland in the neck, consisting of two lobes connected by an isthmus. The thyroid is located at the front of the neck, below the Adam's apple. The thyroid gland secretes thyroid hormones, which primarily influence the metabolic rate and protein synthesis." Therefore, the thyroid plays an important part in weight control. Having something wrong with the thyroid can greatly affect a person's weight or the ability to lose weight.

One of the most noticeable symptoms of hypothyroidism is weight gain and difficulty losing extra weight. The most important step you can do—for weight loss and for your overall health—is to get proper treatment for your thyroid condition. Follow your doctor's instructions. Many doctors will say to consider going gluten-free, cut out sugars and simple carbs, eat plenty of veggies, get some exercise, and take any medication prescribed. Thyroid problems make losing weight difficult, but not impossible. You will require some extra effort and careful planning. You can do what you need to do.

Excuse 186 - I Have a Wheat Intolerance

My daughter Ange is a Certified Holistic Health Practitioner. She does food sensitivity testing. I had her check me and the report came back I had a wheat sensitivity, meaning wheat could be a problem for me. Now sensitivity is a little different from a wheat intolerance. I assume you have had this intolerance diagnosed somehow. Intolerance means your body is really having problems and experiencing poor health symptoms.

Assuming you really have intolerances, I would avoid those

particular foods. You might also have intolerances or allergies to nonfood items as well. You have to consider these sensitivities when you are on your weight loss plan. I saw a program awhile back where the little boy could only eat seven different foods. That's extreme but we live in a society where the food environment is suspect, including pesticides and fertilizers. So no wonder we are seeing more sensitivities, allergies, and intolerances.

You might want to do a sensitivity check, and avoid those foods to which you might be sensitive. After dieting a while, you can check your wellbeing. Many people say they never have felt so well when eliminating sensitive foods. You can always add one back to see if you have unfavorable symptoms. Avoid the bummer foods and eat healthy.

Excuse 187 – All the Other Excuses

I'm sure I only scratched the surface on excuses for not losing your excess weight. So this excuse sums up all those I didn't innumerate. Put your own excuse here and I tell you to stop giving the excuse power over your life and start taking action to help your situation. Whether you go to a clinic, go on a famous diet, or go on a non-diet, the important issue is to stop making excuses and get the weight off that tired body. You can make excuses but you can't lose weight and make excuses.

Chapter 8

Wrap up

Accept or Except No Excuses

"Except" means to "specify as not included in a category or group; exclude." "Accept" means to "consent to receive." So accept means to receive and except means to exclude. So now you have had a grammar lesson, what does grammar have to do with weight loss? Plenty. We are talking about excuses here. As you have seen, there are plenty and I'm sure you could come up with more of them.

I just heard another one yesterday, which went like this. "Everybody is giving me advice, but I know what's best for me." This was from a 600-pound person. I really don't think she knows what's best. Anyway, she is "accepting" her excuses. If you accept an excuse, then you will fail. Somehow, she got out of her excuse place when her doctor told her the next time he'd see her would be when he was filling out her death certificate. She began to reject the excuse and take positive steps about her weight. Hope the delay wasn't too late for her.

In addition, you can't make any excuse exceptions. You can't say I'm going to diet, except I'm not going to stop eating my evening Twinkie. You can't "accept" any excuses, and you can't "except" any. No excuses period.

Zero Excuses

Seems a little impossible—maybe zero is. All we weight-loss dieters let an excuse slip out now and then. However, most of the time we just vent a little steam or wishfully dream of stacks of food. After not eating pizza for months, when you pass a pizza place, you might say wish I could have some pizza. When you get to maintenance level, you will be able to have a piece of pizza, unless you decide pizza is no longer on your healthy eating list. You might be able to make pizza healthier at home.

The closer you can get to zero excuses, the stronger will be your resolve to make your goal no matter what. You will not have any indulgence on Saturday and say I'll hit the diet trail hard again on Monday. It's surprising, well maybe not surprising how often we succumb to an excuse. Sometimes the excuse is almost unconscious or subconscious. That's why we need to guard our thinking when on our weight loss phase, well from now on. Weight loss is hard while weight gain is easy. I can't say I don't ever think excuse, but rarer I put one into practice.

Just another Excuse

Just because you can, doesn't mean you should.

Now since you've lost weight doesn't mean you can totally back off and eat whatever you want. We've tried that before and it doesn't work well. In fact, we gained some weight back. I think we probably used the excuse we could and so we did. Ugh!

Any excuse is not a good excuse, and just because you can, doesn't mean you should. IF you do fall into this temporary sidetrack, shake the monster off, and get back on plan. The regret is not what you *can't* have. The motivation is what you *choose* not to eat right now to reach the better goal of weight loss and better health. Did you notice how easy weight attaches to your body, so let's not use *any excuses*. Carry on with your eating/exercise plan!

Dump the Excuses

When you have a firm hold on your vision of weight loss, don't let distractions, such as excuses, keep you from realizing your vision. Drop the negativity associated with an excuse. If you are walking on the treadmill in the cold of winter, don't say, "I hate this, it's stupid." Review your vision. No more huffing and puffing up the stairs. No more sitting along the path of life and watching everyone jog past you. No, you are working on *your* vision. You have a blessed person in view with many years of exciting life ahead. Keep walking, or as Dora said, keep swimming.

Making excuses is one of the biggest problems to seeing your weight loss goals fulfilled. An excuse is like taking your vision, writing it down, and then drawing an X through it and throwing away the whole dream. You just negated the positive view of yourself and said I can't be that wonderful. You can and you are. Be wonderful to yourself. Your vision is of an amazing person. Don't let excuses bum your progress. Keep seeing yourself as loved, blessed, and resting in grace. Keep your vision free and clear so you can run forward with your dream.

Trash the Excuse and Live

The day you plop the excuse in the garbage, your life begins. Dropping the excuses will change your life. If you have always had a dream to do something but added some excuse, you will never see your dream realized. If you looked at yourself in the mirror and wished you didn't have all the extra weight, has an excuse kept you from achieving your dream?

Your taking action will fulfill many dreams. If you have always wanted to play the guitar nothing will happen unless you get a guitar and take some lessons. Charlene and I both learned to play the guitar many years ago. We needed music for our church services so we bought guitars and took lessons. We even went on to write songs and used them in our church. We could have used excuses that would have kept us from realizing our desire but we didn't.

The same is true for many areas of life. Here we concentrate on weight loss. Change is hard for most people. An excuse will keep you from even trying. Life goes on second by second, minute by minute, and if you don't change now, life will go on by, and you'll have nothing but unfulfilled wishes.

An Excuse Changes Nothing

An excuse is just talk and no action. You complete nothing by exercising an excuse. Now exercising your body will get something done. I'm sure you know people who put on a good talk, but never accomplish anything. They may tell you about all their aches and pains but won't get the weight off causing those aches and pains. This is more than procrastination. This is excusing oneself out of making changes at all. This is procrastination to infinity and beyond. Sounds a little harsh, but excusers need a wakeup bonk or a slap in the back of the head.

If you have no plans to diet, okay fine. Sometimes I come across as saying diet or else. However, this is totally your choice. There is no condemnation if you do or don't go on a weight loss diet. The only issue is making a decision about the weight loss plan and just start. Don't make excuses and do nothing. A decision not to go on a diet is at least making a decision. Then drop the excuses. If you're still making excuses, you haven't made a decision. Maybe you just need to lose the weight.

Don't Lie - No Excuse

Don't add to the world of lies by contributing your excuse. Sounds harsh even as I wrote this. However, an excuse is a self-lie. In most cases, just a lie. Lying has become the "go to" behavior when put to the test. Some people are good liars. Your excuse is either a lie or real. Sometimes you lie to yourself. Sometimes you believe the lie.

When you hear the word "can't" come out of your mouth, you have probably told yourself a lie, even though you actually think you can't. I hear someone say, well I didn't tell a lie I told a fib. Caught in a fib, most people will say they were just joking. The Apostle Paul has this to say, "Do not lie to one another, since you have put off the old man with his deeds" (Colossians 3:9). Life revolves around love. If you love, you don't lie. If you love yourself, you don't lie to yourself. Love comes from Christ in you. When you are tempted to make a lying excuse, stop and say no. I will tell myself the truth.

Excuse Free Zone

I like this phrase—the excuse free zone. Are you living in the excuse free zone? This isn't a place such as a church, or a state, but near you. The excuse free zone should surround you. It's yet another way to say, lose the excuses.

You can so easily excuse your feelings or your actions, or your lack of action. We live in a society where everyone is picking everything apart, particularly what we say. Sometimes you might be better to say nothing. When saying an excuse, better to keep your mouth shut. An excuse is just an explanation for failure. I've been on many diets and they were all failures of which I have excuses.

Some excuses sound legitimate because some are actually true. For example, one diet I went on almost tripled my weekly food budget. I quit the diet. The diet for me was a failure. However, had I continued to spend the money, I might have succeeded, and been broke. Not every diet fits everyone. You will start diets that just don't work for you, even though they might work for someone else. No excuses, in this excuse free zone.

Don't Be a Victim of Excuses

In this book, we are concentrating on the excuses, but there is lots of chat about this problem of being a victim on the internet. Excuses make you a victim. A victim is a person who has been hurt or taken advantage of somehow. Although some people like to be victims—they need help—a victim has lost a chunk of life.

We could talk about life in general and being a victim, but here I want to concentrate on weight. Unfortunately, you are the cause of your overweight condition. Some psychology would say you are the victim and being overweight is not your fault. You are a victim of environment or social injustices. Your family made you fat. As a child, your parents overfed you or fed you unhealthy or fattening foods. In that sense, you are a victim, however, now you have a choice.

The past is past, and excuses about the past do not help. To continue the excuses just adds to your adverse situation. Your excuses keep you from doing what you need to do to get your life into the happy zone. Of course, losing weight isn't going to make you happy if you live by excuses. Begin with getting rid of the excuses, and watch your life bloom.

Excuses or Opportunities

Excuses will always be there for you, but opportunities won't. When we were in Surfside, Florida, we wanted to get up early and watch the sunrise. Everyone said the sunrises were beautiful here. The whole sunrise lasted but minutes and then the sun was up. A few minutes late and we would have missed the beautiful sunrise. Many incidents happen that way in our lives. The door opens, and then closes. Sunrise and sunset, and time marches on.

Sometimes when I write about weight loss, I think I'm writing to the choir. We often struggle with daily weight issues. We allow ourselves to gain some weight, and then we work to get the weight off again. There are stacks of excuses for yo-yo weight gain and loss. I'm certainly not immune to them, but I'm getting better at recognizing them and refusing them more quickly. Today is not yesterday, and tomorrow is not today. We have to live in the now and walk the weight-loss journey of today, Opportunities come and go. Some we can grab some will get away. As one commercial says, "When opportunity knocks, be sure and open the door." Look for opportunities and trash the excuses.

<u>Excuses or Changes</u>

Some people are making excuses and some are making changes. With 95% of weight loss dieters failing, most people are making excuses, and few are making changes. Moreover, the country continues to grow fatter. We know doing the same thing repeatedly, thinking we will get different results, is the definition of insanity. Do you remember Susan Powter and her *Stop the Insanity* diet? We went on her diet. Don't know why we quit, though. She had a good stepper routine we followed. Published back in 1993, I think this idea rang a bell in dieter's heads saying we need to stop all this crazy dieting and get to a plan that works and is healthy.

I don't know how many diets there have been over the years, but all the individual nutritionists and fitness gurus have their diets for individuals. Nevertheless, getting back on topic, we need to scrap the excuses, and make the changes needed to restore our health and take America off the top overweight list. To make progress requires individuals like each of us to make permanent changes.

Weight loss is a choice. An excuse is a choice. Yep. You actually choose to make an excuse. The Bible says out of the heart, the mouth speaks. Some people are excuse minded. Their hearts are negative, and negative comes out in their words. An excuse is a negative phrase, which halts progress. A negative person believes the world owes him or her something. They think if they're having a bad day, everyone else should cater to them. They let their negative feelings and poor attitude drive them on a daily basis. A pessimist is a person who expects the worst. This character trait shows up in every area of life.

In weight loss, being negative comes out as an excuse. What you feed your heart makes a big difference. I say feed you heart with God's Word. One word from God can change your life forever. Once you know who you are according to God, you will grow less negative and more positive about every area of your life. You will become an agent of change, not excuses.

Quit Making Excuses

I love to watch the segment where Bob Newhart as Dr. Switzer is in a counseling session with someone who is terrified someone would bury her alive. After some back and forth conversation, he tells her he can cure her problem. She begins to take notes when He says no need I have just two words to say—"Stop It." This is the "stop it" therapy. Sometimes you just want to shout, "Stop it." I don't want to hear any more excuses. Either lose weight, or don't, but don't give me any excuses for what you decide.

When we were pastors, we would counsel someone and they would give us their tale of woe, we would counter with what they needed to do. Did they do what we suggested—no! Doctors believe 50 - 75% of their patients don't take their prescribed medication. Our daughter talks with clients about their eating issues and gives them a plan to overcome. Do they follow the plan? Maybe a few, but to her consternation, most don't. Do whatever you want to do, but quit making excuses for your bad decisions. I'm a proponent of the "stop it" therapy. When an excuse begins to form in your mouth, don't go there. Stop it.

Write Down Your Excuses and Then Tear Them Up

If you are having trouble with excuses, then you need to make some changes. In my opinion, an excuse is a mental coping mechanism to help you excuse your failure. No one likes to fail. An excuse helps you hide your failures. At least in your thinking. An excuse becomes a rational reason excusing the failure, thus lessening the blow.

If you are struggling with weight loss, perhaps your excuses are to blame. My suggestion would be to sit down in a quiet place and have a heart to heart talk with yourself. What excuses are you making which have hindered your progress in life and specifically your weight loss goals? Write them down. Ask the Lord to help erase these excuses from your life. Then tear up the paper and throw it away symbolically saying, I'm not going to make these excuses anymore.

Put the excuse thinking out of your mind. Become solution minded. Don't see life as one failure after another. See yourself as a winner. Look for the good. Change the old patterns in your life into new patterns of success. Look for your success each day. You ate on plan today. You are a winner. No more excuses, please.

<u>There Is No Such Thing As Can't</u>

On one episode of *The Biggest Loser,* the theme was "I can't lose weight on my own." Since this was no excuses season for the contestants, two points came to mind.

First, how difficult do you find losing weight on your own. There is no one to push you and no one to encourage you. Most of us struggle with motivation, such as hard to get motivated to work out. Most people don't like to go for a walk alone. Many dieters will give up with this excuse.

There are ways to overcome this thinking. The easiest way is not trying this alone. Walk with someone or walk your dog. Go to a gym where you have others around you or get a trainer to push you. Join a website and get involved. Join a club like a hiking club or a workout club. There are many ways to keep from being alone.

Second, get rid of the words "I can't" from your vocabulary. You can't if you say you can't. You can if you say you can. This is more than positive thinking or positive confession—which are important. Your words release the power to overcome. "Can't" just sounds defeating. The word removes the desire or will to succeed in your weight loss efforts. Without any "will" you certainly deplete the ability to win.

Yes, we know the difficulty in losing alone. Losing is hard whether you are alone or not. However, weight loss is not impossible. In fact, very possible. Search out ways to lose the weight on your own. Don't let "can't" seep into your thinking. You can. Yes, you can.

Accept the responsibility

"That means I took liberty to eat anything I pleased and refused to accept responsibility for my actions. It's one thing to admit a problem, but it's quite another to own it." Scott Davis. Most of us overweight or obese people have a problem owning up to the situation we find ourselves. In other words, accepting the fact, I'm fat and accepting the responsibility is mine for getting fat.

Many people admit to the problem and make changes. However, most believe why I can't lose weight is someone else's fault or something else. Maybe you are in a low-income family and have to visit food pantries, only getting what they give you. You have to do what you have to do. Even then, you don't have to overeat. Eat a few less baked beans and thank God for the blessing of beans.

Maybe you had a traumatic event occur in your life. There's where the Lord's strength and grace comes in to get you through without thinking eating will resolve the issue. Cast your care on Him and take responsibility for you weight. There is never a good excuse. You *can* overcome.

Diet Bumps - No Excuses

So what's your excuse? Are you waiting for Monday, next week or the New Year? Hey, you talking to me? About what am I talking or writing? I'm talking about excuses.

"Ninety-nine percent of the failures come from people who have the habit of making excuses." George Washington Carver

Excuses are failures. We have enough failures but we don't have to add to them by using excuses. Course we can excuse our failures. Excuses hurt us more than anyone else.

When we went to school, if we were sick we had to bring an excuse from home. The note from mom justified why we were absent. One of our parents had to sign the note to legitimize the excuse. We learned to try excuses early in our life. The dog ate my homework. I had to go to church Wednesday night with my parents. The more we worked at excuses the better we got.

Do we really fool ourselves by making up an excuse? Excuses diminish our life each time we say one. We could have exercised, could have become fit, but we just excused it away. Excuses are for the lazy. Excuses are for those who just watch life pass by with no participation in the joys life has to offer.

"People want a cop-out, listen I'm a realist and I talk about motivation, talk about all the things it takes to be greater or are important to win and people want to use excuses all the time." Mike Ditka.

If we want to win the war of weight loss, we can't make excuses. I like the saying, "No excuses." When the game is over, I don't want to have to make excuses for losing. I want to win. No Excuses.

You're Stronger than Any Excuse

Excuses can be habit-forming. It's easy to give an excuse for why you haven't lost the weight you need to lose. Excuses come easy. The more you make excuses, the harder it is to stop making excuses. Excuses are like the annoying pesky fly buzzing around you. Many just put up with an excuse. You may swat at it a couple of times yet the little booger still pesters you. Does the excuse become annoying?

You are stronger than your excuses. In fact, you are more than a conqueror through Christ. Romans 8:37 adds, "In all these things."

means in dieting and making excuses about your failures. You do have the power to quit the excuses. You are stronger than your excuses. You can conquer every one of them. In the flesh not so easy. However, through Christ, you can defeat every foe, including excuses. Therefore, when you are tempted to make an excuse, grab hold of the promise you are more than this excuse. You are a conqueror, yes, and more than a conqueror. You are stronger than any excuse.

If you are serious you'll find a way; if not you will find an excuse

There are two types of people. There are the excuse makers and the way makers. What inventions would we have today an excuse would have destroyed? Edison could have said can't and none of his inventions would have developed into reality. Maybe you have food allergies, budget restraints, or any of a million obstacles facing a weight loss journey. Instead of letting them be an excuse, seek to find a way over, around, or through them. There are solutions to problems. I like Tony Robbins quote, "Stay committed to your decisions, but stay *flexible* in your approach."

Have a strong core reason why you want to lose weight. However, you may need some flexibility in how you reach your goals. Everyday things change. Schedules change. Mood and emotions change. Finances change. Life fills the days with change, which requires flexibility and problem solving. There will be a way but you may have to look for it. We have an internet where we can find all kinds of helpful information. There are alternates to recipes and foods as well as ways to enjoy the weight loss journey. Find the way and lose the excuse.

Start your no excuses diet today. Make your weight loss journey your way of life and enjoy your fat free days ahead.

<u>Are Your Excuses Stronger Than Your Dreams</u>

Here is a definition of a dream you can put to the test: *A dream is an inspiring picture of the future that energizes your mind, will and emotions, empowering you to do everything you can to achieve it.* A dream worth pursuing is a picture and blueprint of a person's purpose and potential. As Sharon Hull says, "A dream is the seed of possibility planted in the soul of a human being, which calls him to pursue a unique path to the realization of his purpose."

I would like to add to that definition the source of your dream. Great dreams are God inspired. Some might say it was a calling or a vision. Though this applies to all of life, what is your vision of your weight and health? Is your dream to travel, see the sights, and visit special locations? You don't have to have big dreams, which have no basis in your reality. They could be goals, ambitions, or desires. Is your dream fading with age? Is your dream stronger than any excuse you might have to reach the unreachable star? Can you see yourself the weight you desire and is that dream strong enough to take you there? The best is yet to come.

About The Author

Jack G Elder graduated from Ashland High School in Ashland, Oregon. He received an AA degree in Electronics from Oregon Tech. He received a Bachelor of Theology degree from Melodyland School of Theology, a Masters of Divinity, Doctor of Theology, and Doctor of Ministry degrees from Christian International. He worked for IBM for 31 years and Heidelberg another 13 years. He was a bi-vocational pastor in churches in both Southern California and Georgia. He and his wife, Charlene, began JubileeOnlineChurch.org—A Church without Walls Sharing God's Grace and Love, their website where you can read their daily devotions. You can also go to JubileeHealthPlace.org and read his diet and health articles. See JackandCharlene.com for all their books. He is a proud husband, father, grandfather, and great-grandfather. He enjoys writing, teaching, blogging, hiking, traveling, and playing games.